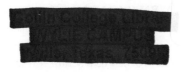

Expert Clinician to
Novice Nurse Educator

Jeanne Merkle Sorrell, PhD, RN, FAAN, is professor emerita of nursing at George Mason University, where she taught for over 20 years in the BSN, MSN, and PhD programs, as well as serving in various administrative roles. After moving to Cleveland, Ohio, she worked as a senior nurse scientist in the Office of Nursing Research and Innovation at the Cleveland Clinic. She is currently a contributing faculty member at Walden University.

Dr. Sorrell earned a BSN from the University of Michigan, an MSN from the University of Wisconsin, and a PhD from George Mason University. Her scholarly interests focus on philosophical inquiry, writing across the curriculum, qualitative research, and ethical considerations for patients with chronic illness. In addition to research on the role of novice nurse educators, she has used interpretive phenomenology to explore ethical concerns in the lived experience of patients and caregivers with Alzheimer's disease. Findings from the research were presented in a video, *Quality Lives: Ethics in the Care of Persons With Alzheimer's*, and a play, *Six Characters in Search of an Answer*, both of which received Sigma Theta Tau International Media Awards. She is co-author of a book with her daughter, Christine Dinkins, *Our Dissertations, Ourselves: Shared Stories of Women's Dissertation Journeys*.

Pamela R. Cangelosi, PhD, RN, CNE, ANEF, is the associate dean for academics and a professor at Shenandoah University, Winchester, Virginia. She has over 25 years of teaching experience and has taught classroom and clinical courses for all levels of nurses—from practical (LPN) to doctoral nursing students. Her clinical area of expertise is primarily in medical–surgical nursing.

Dr. Cangelosi earned her diploma in practical nursing from the Loudoun County School of Practical Nursing, an ADN and BSN from Shenandoah College, an MSN from Marymount University, and a PhD in nursing from George Mason University. Dr. Cangelosi's research has focused on the education of nontraditional nursing students, especially RN to BSN and accelerated second-degree students, faculty, and programs. She has also concentrated her research on clinical nurse educators and their preparation for clinical teaching. Findings from her research have been presented at national and international professional conferences and published in the leading professional nursing education journals.

Expert Clinician to Novice Nurse Educator

Learning From First-Hand Narratives

Jeanne Merkle Sorrell, PhD, RN, FAAN
Pamela R. Cangelosi, PhD, RN, CNE, ANEF

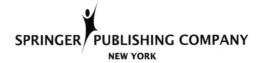

SPRINGER PUBLISHING COMPANY
NEW YORK

Springer Publishing Company, LLC
11 West 42nd Street
New York, NY 10036
www.springerpub.com

Acquisitions Editor: Joseph Morita
Production Editor: Kris Parrish
Composition: MPS Limited

ISBN: 978-0-8261-2598-9
e-book ISBN: 978-0-8261-2599-6

15 16 17 18 19 / 5 4 3 2 1

The author and the publisher of this Work have made every effort to use sources believed to be reliable to provide information that is accurate and compatible with the standards generally accepted at the time of publication. Because medical science is continually advancing, our knowledge base continues to expand. Therefore, as new information becomes available, changes in procedures become necessary. We recommend that the reader always consult current research and specific institutional policies before performing any clinical procedure. The author and publisher shall not be liable for any special, consequential, or exemplary damages resulting, in whole or in part, from the readers' use of, or reliance on, the information contained in this book. The publisher has no responsibility for the persistence or accuracy of URLs for external or third-party Internet websites referred to in this publication and does not guarantee that any content on such websites is, or will remain, accurate or appropriate.

Library of Congress Cataloging-in-Publication Data
Sorrell, Jeanne Merkle, author.
  Expert clinician to novice nurse educator : learning from first-hand narratives /
Jeanne Merkle Sorrell, Pamela Rubel Cangelosi.
    p. ; cm.
  Includes bibliographical references and index.
  ISBN 978-0-8261-2598-9 — ISBN 978-0-8261-2599-6 (ebook)
  I. Cangelosi, Pamela Rubel, author. II. Title.
  [DNLM: 1. Faculty, Nursing—Personal Narratives. 2. Education, Nursing—Personal Narratives.
3. Nurse Clinicians—education—Personal Narratives. 4. Teaching—Personal Narratives. WY 19.1]
  RT86.4
  610.7306′9—dc23
                                                                          2015019436

Special discounts on bulk quantities of our books are available to corporations, professional associations, pharmaceutical companies, health care organizations, and other qualifying groups. If you are interested in a custom book, including chapters from more than one of our titles, we can provide that service as well.

For details, please contact:
Special Sales Department, Springer Publishing Company, LLC
11 West 42nd Street, 15th Floor, New York, NY 10036-8002
Phone: 877-687-7476 or 212-431-4370; Fax: 212-941-7842
E-mail: sales@springerpub.com

Printed in the United States of America by Gasch Printing.

To the talented and patient clinical nurse educators who continue to guide learning for new nurses.

Contents

Part II. Teaching Thinking

Part III. Learning From First-Hand Narratives

Part IV. Storied Reflections

Contributors

Christine Sorrell Dinkins, PhD (Chapter 6)
Associate Professor of Philosophy
Wofford College
Spartanburg, South Carolina

Felicia Michelle Glasgow, EdD, MNSc, RN, LNC (Chapter 8)
Professor of Nursing
Central Texas College
Killeen, Texas

Lorena Jung, PhD, RN (Chapter 7)
Assistant Professor of Nursing
Shenandoah University
Winchester, Virginia

Meggen Platzar, BSN, RN, CMSRN (Chapter 9)
Clinical Instructor, Office of Nursing Education and Professional
    Development
Cleveland Clinic Health System
Cleveland, Ohio

Preface

I am buckling my seatbelt to explore the educator's role.
It is a short distance ride. However, the next ride could possibly
be with an educator in the driver's seat—my seatbelt will still be
needed. But I will further investigate to ascertain other items
to take on the trip.

—Melody

The nurse educator role often looks deceptively simple. Compared to the complexity of bedside care for a patient with multiple comorbidities and hour-by-hour monitoring, watching over students to guide their learning may appear easy. Yet, when experienced nurse clinicians try out this new endeavor for the first time, they often describe themselves as frustrated and uncertain about how to best implement the role. Through years of experience as clinicians, nurses often arrive at a comfort zone where they know what to do for their patients in order to keep them safe and enhance their healing. When moving to the nurse educator role, however, many of the usual guidelines for practice may no longer seem relevant.

Nursing education today is faced with many challenges. The need for education of more nurses, the increasing numbers of individuals who want to enter nursing education programs, and the shortage of nursing faculty to teach these aspiring students have raised new questions about how best to prepare the nursing workforce for the present and future. A January 2014 report by the U.S. Bureau of Labor Statistics estimated that employment of registered nurses will grow by 19% between 2012 and 2022—faster than the average for all other occupations (Bureau of Labor Statistics, U.S. Department of Labor, 2014). A need for over 1 million new nurses is projected for 2022 (Robert Wood Johnson Foundation, 2014). This increased demand for nurses is due to a variety of factors. People are living longer and older people often have more medical problems than younger people, creating a need for nurses to educate and care for more persons with various chronic illnesses. In addition, nurses will be needed to care for the increased numbers of individuals who will have access to health care services as a result of the 2010 Patient Protection and Affordable Care Act. Also, financial pressure on hospitals to discharge patients as quickly as possible is likely to create a need for more nurses to care for patients at home or in long-term care centers.

How are schools of nursing going to accommodate these new nurse applicants? There is a critical shortage of nursing faculty, which limits the number of students who can be enrolled at a time when the need for nurses is growing quickly. In a report by the American Association of Colleges of Nursing (AACN), *2013–2014 Enrollment and Graduations in Baccalaureate and Graduate Programs in Nursing*, almost two thirds of respondents cited faculty shortages as the reason for not accepting all qualified applicants. The report revealed that 79,089 qualified applicants were denied admission to U.S. baccalaureate and graduate nursing programs in 2012 because of insufficient numbers of faculty, clinical sites, classroom space, clinical preceptors, and budget constraints (AACN, 2014). A lack of nursing faculty is also an international problem, with qualified student applicants turned away in such countries as Canada, China, Australia, and Malaysia (Reid, Hinderer, Jarosinski, Mister, & Seldomridge, 2013).

Although accrediting agencies call for nursing faculty educated with a graduate degree, this is difficult in today's health care climate. Nurses with doctorates still comprise less than 1% of the U.S. population. Increasing numbers of nurses are pursuing graduate education, but the job market for these nurses is growing faster than jobs for RNs, meaning that schools of nursing that want to hire faculty with a graduate degree are competing with the 50,000 new positions projected for nurse anesthetists, certified nurse midwives, and nurse practitioners—all of which usually come with a much higher salary than nurse educators receive (Robert Wood Johnson Foundation, 2014).

With both nursing education programs and clinical agencies stretched to the maximum to meet the needs of their institutions, there is an immediate need for creative options to increase the supply of competent nurse educators who can effectively teach vital clinical skills to future nurses. Experienced nurse clinicians offer a valuable option. Yet, they are often asked to function as clinical nurse educators with little or no education for the role. They may receive an orientation to their assigned hospital but, for the most part, are left to themselves to figure out how to teach. Some of them find a way through their frustrations to become effective faculty. Many, however, give up in frustration and return to their previous clinical role. This not only leaves the aspiring nurse educator with a feeling of failure, but also negatively affects nursing programs that may be critically short of clinical faculty.

As the nursing faculty shortage grows, more nurse clinicians are going to find themselves working with students, either as adjunct faculty or hospital preceptors. Too often, these novice nurse educators are on a journey without readable signposts. How do you keep the patient safe while allowing the student nurse to practice doing something for that patient for the first time? If some students are slow to catch on to what seems simple to you, how long should you wait before you fail them? If you let weak students continue in the nursing program, at some point, one of them may unwittingly harm a patient. But if a student fails, do you have enough evidence that, given enough time, the student would have been able to pull the pieces of a puzzle together and become a competent and caring nurse?

First-hand narratives in this book from nurse clinicians, faculty, and students explore questions like these. All of the narratives are from qualitative research studies. We are nurse educators who taught together in a graduate nursing program designed to prepare nurse educators. Stories in Chapters 1, 2, 4, and 5 were collected during 4 years of a successful Clinical Nurse Educator Academy that we initiated to address the need to prepare experienced clinicians for new roles as clinical nurse educators. Stories in Chapter 3 are from a qualitative research study that was implemented with nursing students who described caring and uncaring experiences with clinical nurse educators. This chapter also includes stories from research studies on cultural diversity and bullying. Chapter 6 focuses on aspects of the clinical educator role related to critical and ethical thinking. Chapters 7, 8, and 9 contain reflections of nurse educators looking back on their first teaching experiences in a school of nursing or hospital. Finally, Chapter 10 discusses strategies for clinical nurse educators to use in addressing recommendations by the study, *Educating Nurses: A Call for Radical Transformation* (Benner, Sutphen, Leonard, & Day, 2010). Some participants from the Clinical Nurse Educator Academy also share their thoughts after an 8-year journey from their original exposure to the nurse educator role.

Information in these chapters is intended to apply to clinical nurse educators teaching new nurse graduates, as well as nursing students. For readability, however, the term "student" is often used to refer to either a new graduate nurse or student nurse since they are both "students" of the nurse educator. Pseudonyms are used for all of the research participants whose stories are included here but the stories are exactly as told to the researchers. In carrying out the research, we found that the journey of assuming a new role as clinical nurse educator is only partly explained by the actual "how to" course work that nurses may receive during their formal education. Participants described unexpected challenges and transformations in their own identity and relationships that are a vital part of learning a new professional role.

The quote at the beginning of this preface from Melody, a participant in the Clinical Nurse Educator Academy and an expert clinician, illustrates the mix of both excitement and anxiety that novice educators often face. We wanted to write this book because we have seen clinicians struggling with transitioning to this new clinical educator role. As several of the research participants commented, many nurses take on the clinical educator role without the opportunity to explore with faculty and peers what to expect in the role and how to implement it effectively. This book illustrates the difficulties of moving into a new role as a novice, offering perspectives of a diverse group of participants who lived with the experience and learned. The book is not designed to be a step-by-step prescription in how to implement the clinical educator role but, instead, a stimulus to engage aspiring or new clinical educators in thinking about situations they may encounter and to help them transition to their new role. Nurse educators already practicing in that role may also find that the stories help them to think about the challenges and wonderful benefits of being a clinical nurse educator.

Stories in this book show how clinical nurse educators make an important difference for students and new graduates. Many of the stories were told through tears, as research participants remembered how someone stepped in at a critical time to help or to reassure them that they had done well for their patient. But, there are also stories about faculty or colleagues who failed to support them in their learning. And, faculty themselves share insights into what they wish they had done differently to guide students in their learning.

Stories are an important way of capturing the narratives of our lives. In Barry Lopez's book, *Crow and Weasel*, Badger states, "If stories come to you, care for them. And learn to give them away where they are needed" (Lopez, 1990, p. 48). The stories in this book speak of common experiences, emotions, and challenges faced by students, new graduates, and faculty across different nursing programs and different clinical specialties. The stories give voice to the challenges and opportunities inherent in the clinical nurse educator role. We hope that this book will be read by both new and experienced nurse educators who may gain support, perspective, insight, inspiration, and guidance from stories of those who struggled to make a difference in learning for their students.

Jeanne Merkle Sorrell
Pamela R. Cangelosi

REFERENCES

American Association of Colleges of Nursing. (2014). Nursing faculty shortage fact sheet. Retrieved from www.aacn.nche.edu/media-relations/Faculty ShortageFS.pdf

Benner, P., Sutphen, M., Leonard, V., & Day, L. (2010). *Educating nurses: A call for radical transformation.* San Francisco, CA: Jossey-Bass.

Bureau of Labor Statistics, U.S. Department of Labor. (2014). *Registered nurses. Occupational outlook handbook, 2014–2015 edition.* Retrieved from www.bls .gov/ooh/healthcare/registered-nurses.htm#tab-6

Lopez, B. (1990). *Crow and Weasel.* San Francisco, CA: North Point Press.

Reid, T. P., Hinderer, K. A., Jarosinski, J. M., Mister, B. J., & Seldomridge, L. A. (2013). Expert clinician to clinical teacher: Developing a faculty academy and mentoring initiative. *Nurse Education in Practice, 13*, 288–293.

Robert Wood Johnson Foundation. (2014). Nursing job outlook sunny as experts project need for more than one million new nurses by 2022. Retrieved from www.rwjf.org/en/about-rwjf/newsroom/newsroom-content/2014/05/long-term-job-outlook-for-nurses-is-sunny--as-experts-project-na.html

Acknowledgments

We gratefully acknowledge the many persons who have contributed to the completion of this book through their advice and support. The qualitative research studies reported here were supported by funding from the National League for Nursing and the George Mason University College of Nursing and Health Science. Research colleagues in the Office of Nursing Research and Innovation at the Cleveland Clinic offered valuable support in the planning of the book. We especially want to acknowledge our wise and patient husbands, Gregory Sorrell and Frank Cangelosi, for their always-ready support; our participants, who trusted us to share their stories of struggles and research; and each other, for the shared journey from teacher/student to friends and co-authors, as we continue to learn from each other.

PART I

The Journey From Clinician to Educator

CHAPTER 1

Moving From an "Expert" to a "Novice" Role

The concept of expert to novice is not new to me. In part, because
I have had so many roles in nursing. I like to challenge myself and
try something new. Each time I try something new, it is with angst
that I am, once again, a novice!

—Jill

In response to the nursing shortage, many schools of nursing have increased recruitment and enrollment of nursing students (Culleiton & Shellenbarger, 2007). Although this is necessary to meet the increasing health care needs of today's society, it seriously exacerbates the ongoing nursing faculty shortage. Lecture-style classrooms may be able to accommodate more students with less impact on faculty numbers; however, clinical teaching and some of the more learner-focused active methods of teaching that are becoming increasingly more popular in nursing classrooms require a higher faculty-to-student ratio. Depending on the clinical setting, the clinical agency policies, and the respective state board of nursing mandates, faculty-to-student ratios in the clinical setting can range from 1:15 to 1:6, and even 1:1 in a preceptor model of instruction. Unfortunately, as the numbers of nursing students increase, the numbers of nursing faculty may not. The aging faculty who are close to retirement, the lower salaries in academia, and an insufficient pool of potential nurse educators in graduate programs (American Association of Colleges of Nursing, 2014) are all cited as factors in the ever increasing shortage of qualified nursing faculty.

At present, nursing schools are attempting to expand their programs to accommodate the increasing numbers of applicants required to fill the over 1 million new nursing positions that projections indicate will be needed by 2022 (Robert Wood Johnson Foundation, 2014). At the same time, hospitals are struggling with how to address the "preparation-to-practice" gap that has been identified. New graduate nurses constitute over 10% of the nursing staff for a typical hospital and this number is certain to increase in the future. A national survey of schools of nursing and hospitals showed that although 90% of nursing faculty believe that their graduates are prepared to provide safe and effective care, 90% of hospital-based educators are questioning the practice readiness of new nurse graduates (Nurse Executive Center, 2008). Thus, many hospitals are implementing nurse residency programs in an effort to accelerate practice readiness of new graduates. Experienced nurse clinicians at these institutions will be called on to serve as clinical educators for these new nurses.

Many of these expert clinicians have not yet experienced what it is like to teach and find themselves, once again, a novice. They may have a bachelor's, master's, or doctoral degree, but no experience or formal preparation in teaching and learning (Anderson, 2009; Schriner, 2007). Benner (1982) has characterized a novice nurse as a beginner who must have rules to guide practice, because there is no experience from which to draw conclusions. The rules, however, are context-free, so that the novice does not know which rules are most relevant in a real situation or when an exception to the rule should be considered. This type of discretionary judgment is developed through experience. Thus, it is important to identify ways to enhance competency and confidence of expert clinicians as they move into a new educator role.

THE STORIES

Nursing history is rich in stories, but a focus on the science of nursing has sometimes obscured the stories of real life experiences that can teach us so much. In an effort to address the need for mentoring of new clinical faculty, the authors designed and implemented a Clinical Nurse Educator Academy to prepare experienced clinicians for new roles as part-time or full-time clinical nurse educators (Cangelosi, Crocker, & Sorrell, 2009). Through written narratives, 32 nurse clinicians shared their perspectives as they prepared for new roles as clinical nurse educators. This chapter presents stories focused on participants' responses to the following interview prompt:

> Think about what it is like to move from a role as an "expert" to a "novice." Describe an incident that reflects your concerns about moving from the clinician to the clinical nurse educator role.

Jill's comment at the opening of this chapter reflects the essence of other participants' comments: Moving to a new role as clinical nurse educator left the nurse clinician once again feeling like a novice. The participants, however, did not see the novice role as negative, but rather a time for them to learn new skills. Although being a novice was described as being "unsettling," "uncomfortable," and causing "mixed feelings," these participants embraced the chance to be a novice again and forward their career goals.

Embracing the Novice

April clearly verbalized the benefits she realized from being a novice:

> I have been a nurse for 32 years. I have been a novice many times. I have been an expert a few times. … Being a novice makes me feel young. … I allow myself to be a novice, to not know everything and to learn from others and the job itself.

Anne shared her feelings about why she embarked on the transitional journey toward the role of clinical nurse educator:

> The most memorable events in my career of feeling good about making a difference have been the times I had to hold my breath, put fear aside, and dive right in!

Veronica described how she realized that putting herself in the role of "student" again was providing her with important new skills and self-confidence:

> I absorbed all of what had just happened, and I processed what it all meant to me. Suddenly, I felt rejuvenated—and free. I didn't have to be the Perfect Teacher. I could make mistakes. And moreover, I could make those mistakes in front of everyone, and it would still be okay.

Susan described her reflections about putting herself in the role of a novice so frequently, coming to the conclusion that it was the right thing for her:

> I did have an "a-ha" moment or personal epiphany today when I realized that by trying on many nursing-related hats throughout my professional career, I often keep myself at the level of novice—not always, but often enough to note this. What is that about? Does it protect me from assuming responsibility? I don't think so, since most of my positions have been in management, and I seem to always rise to a leadership role of some kind. Still, I think it's important for me to consider the possible secondary gain in frequently returning to the level of novice. Or am I just a lifelong learner who is not uncomfortable in the role of novice?
>
> I have played a lot of roles, and learned a lot along the way, including how to become very good at most of my jobs, which means that I have learned how to learn, or at least how I learn best. Isn't this the point of the journey in the first place? If one is not learning, not growing, one is stagnating, or worse. I am passionate about lifelong learning, for myself, and encourage it in others. ...But in order to learn, one must start at a position of incompetency, which can be very uncomfortable, and for many adults, intolerable. This is why people stop learning. They can't stand exposing the fact that they don't know something. If you can stand to feel temporarily and

situationally incompetent, the world can teach you so many things!

Eileen described how being a novice again had helped her understand how her students may feel. This gave her a great deal of personal and professional satisfaction:

> I had forgotten how anxious students are about accomplishing simple tasks. I was forced to begin thinking about nursing from the novice point of view. The observations and conclusions made on a daily basis by seasoned nurses are not something that can be taught in a 4-hour clinical. … If we put ourselves in the place of the student and remember what it was like for us, we have an opportunity to make a huge difference in a student nurse's professional journey.

Ellyn also reflected on what had helped her when she was first a novice nurse and how she now wanted to help others love the nursing profession:

> We all must remember that we also were novices once. Those who took the time to nurture and mentor us have done us a great service; moreover, they are the reason why we stuck it out through rough times and helped us to learn to love the nursing profession.

Although it was clear that participants appreciated the necessity of feeling like a novice as they transitioned to the nurse educator role, they also faced this transition with a mix of excitement and anxiety. The theme "leaving my comfort zone" that emerged from analysis of the research interviews illustrates these ambivalent feelings.

"Leaving My Comfort Zone"

Joanie described how it was difficult to leave her comfort zone to enter an area where she was a novice again, but she knew it was an excellent opportunity, even though she still had considerable fear about it. Her detailed reflection is included here because it captures the ambivalence about the transition to the novice role that so many of the participants seemed to feel:

> Advancing in my clinical nursing career was a process
> that was gradual, unassuming, and rather comfortable.
> I worked as a newly graduated nurse in med–surg (because
> that's what one usually did in the '70s), and then switched
> to a specialty area. Over a span of 28 years, I became
> increasingly competent and proficient in the pediatric
> and newborn arena. I climbed the clinical ladder as far as
> I could go. I became certified in my field and was consid-
> ered somewhat of an expert. With ever-increasing knowl-
> edge, experience, and confidence, I felt accomplished,
> credible, and well respected. All was right with the world!
> Why would I upset this perfectly stocked apple cart?
>
> When another opportunity became available, however,
> I decided to leave my comfort zone and forge ahead. This
> was a scary proposition for me, however, because this par-
> ticular opportunity wouldn't have me advancing at the
> bedside and this didn't follow the natural progression of
> my career path. Woe is me!
>
> I thought that I had a fairly good grasp of what the job
> entailed.... I was pumped and excited to get those new
> nurses assigned to good preceptors, to orient students to the
> NICU [neonatal intensive care unit] and to do the best that
> I could in this new role. Although I was definitely a begin-
> ner in this new role when I started almost 4 years ago, and
> received only minimal orientation, I wasn't too apprehensive
> and felt that if I came upon an unfamiliar situation I could
> probably "just wing it." I had a positive attitude, good inten-
> tions, and support from management. Plus, it meant a pay
> raise and no holiday/weekend requirements. This might just
> work out fine. And then I had my "a-ha" moment.
>
> Shortly after starting this new position, I took a trip to
> California and brought along some nursing journals to read
> in the plane. I don't remember which particular state we
> were flying over at the time, but I do remember that I was in
> the plane when I read something that really gave me a jolt. It
> was an article about clinical experiences for nursing students

and the responsibilities of both student and instructor. The student is owed (and deserves) an instructor, preceptor, and/or unit facilitator, who is well versed and properly educated on evidence-based methods regarding knowledge acquisition, effective teaching strategies, and supportive relationship building. The "new" and "old" hires merit someone who understands how psychomotor and social skills are acquired and enhanced and where each person is on their career journey. Good intentions can only go so far.

I knew then that although I had many years of life and career experience, I was a mere babe in the area of staff and student development. I also realized that I must further my formal education and keep current on issues related to this new endeavor because that is what is owed to those whom I support and orient. Hopefully, I have become increasingly competent, proficient, and credible in this new role. However, I don't think that I ever will (or should) become too comfortable in this position. There is too much at stake for that to happen.

The fact that Joanie remembers so vividly, 4 years later, her "a-ha" moment, when she realized with a jolt the career change that she was about to launch, suggests the impact that this career change has on experienced clinicians comfortable in their work. As noted in the preface, another participant in the study, Melody, also anticipated challenges ahead and was buckling her seatbelt in preparation:

I am buckling my seatbelt to explore the educator's role. It is a short distance ride. However, the next ride could possibly be with an educator in the driver's seat—my seatbelt will still be needed. But, I will further investigate to ascertain other items to take on the trip.

Most of the participants in the study received very little formal preparation before they began their new role. Fiona described how she had to plunge in without much help on her first day as a nurse educator, figuring things out on her own:

The call was a plea to work on a medical–surgical floor with a group of students in their last clinical rotation.

The regular instructor had become seriously ill and was no longer able to work. After depleting all of the reasons I could not accept the offer, I finally agreed. I was told where to go, when to go—and that a contract would be forthcoming. I was instructed to assign these students to patients and to oversee their performance. I was reassured that it would be an easy assignment and that I would be fine. The regular faculty was a phone call away and would check on me. That was the beginning of my adjunct career and the extent of my mentorship for that clinical rotation. I was given a list of clinical objectives and an evaluation sheet for each student and the rest was up to me. The visit from the mentor never occurred.

Fiona reflected further on her realization of the importance of the nurse educator role and the responsibility that ensued with accepting this role:

If I could only use one word to describe my move from a role as a clinician to a nurse educator, it would have to be fear. ... I don't believe I had any idea of what a full-time educator's role was. ... I had been transformed from a very autonomous home health nurse to a scared rabbit. The realization that I was now responsible for educating the nurses of the future—the very nurses who would probably be taking care of *me*—hit home.

In summary, it was clear from participants' stories that they were excited about becoming a novice again because they would gain new skills that they could use to share their extensive clinical knowledge with students. At the same time, however, this transition into the novice role created fear and stress, especially because most of them got little to no formal preparation for their new role. The sense of responsibility that came with the clinical nurse educator position only added to the stress.

All of the stories from participants illustrated how transitioning from the expert clinician to the nurse educator role caused the participants to reflect on their strengths and weaknesses, successes and problems in the transition process. Veronica's description of her transition into a preceptor role captures the feelings and emotions that can come with this role change. She was excited at the opportunity to share her knowledge with others, but found the transition road a rocky one. She tells her story with brutal honesty and an engaging sense of humor:

Shakespeare once wrote, "The fool thinks himself to be wise, but the wise man knows himself to be a fool." When I first became a preceptor on my labor, delivery, and recovery unit, I thought myself very wise indeed. My 2½ years of experience put me worlds ahead of my newly graduated preceptee, Kathy, and I was ready to bestow upon her the treasure trove of my knowledge. By the end of that preceptorship, and more so with each preceptorship I take on, I found myself squarely fixed in the humble seat of "student," and I learned an important lesson: The more you teach, the more you learn you have to learn.

When I took on Kathy, I intended to teach quite a bit. I was going to teach her the essentials of labor and delivery, to be sure, but I was also going to teach my coworkers what a great and knowledgeable nurse I was. It would take some hindsight to see, but I was also trying to inculcate in myself a sense that I was, in fact, a capable and intelligent nurse. It wasn't really about Kathy. It was about me.

Throughout that semester, I attached myself to Kathy's hip, ready to pounce on any teaching opportunity, and prepared to catch any mistake that she made. As it turned out, Kathy, who had completed a nurse internship the previous summer, was already quite capable. In fact, her preceptor the previous summer had taught her much of the essentials that she needed to know. I steamed, shuffled my shoes, and pondered: Surely there must be something I could teach her. I mean, after two-and-a-half years of nursing, I must be smarter than she is…right?

Over the next 10 weeks, I bombarded Kathy with articles to read, protocols to memorize, and pop quizzes over which to hurdle. At first, she obliged me. Then she ignored me. But soon, after 8 weeks, Kathy fired me.

I'll never forget the call I got from the new hire coordinator, Judy. She said that Kathy had come to her and said that, although I was, she assured Judy, a very good teacher, she felt that, personality-wise, we just didn't mesh that well. Kathy had offered that, since she and a coworker of mine, Doris, got on so well that one day I was sick and Doris had taken on Kathy, perhaps Doris and I could share Kathy as our orientee?

I was disappointed, baffled, and completely humiliated. Here, I had built myself up to be the Ultimate Preceptor, a Great Nurse Educator in the making, yet I had gotten fired from my first job. I was a failure, and everyone on the unit would know it, but most of all, I would know it.

I learned a very important lesson from that experience: Precepting is not about me; it's about the person I am with. Absorbing Jean Watson's theory, I learned that we—myself and my orientee—are partners in the teaching–learning process: that I can offer her helpful knowledge, and she can offer me helpful knowledge. We are both teachers, and we are both learners. Moreover, it's not just about what I want to teach. It's about what the orientee wants and needs to learn. Every teaching–learning experience has to be tailored to that person, or else, for that person, it will be impersonal, irrelevant, and ignored.

Since Kathy, I've had two wonderful precepting experiences. … Every student has been different, and every one has taught me so much. Hopefully, I've taught them something, too! But in the end, I'm not so much teaching them, I think, as helping them to achieve what they latently have the ability to achieve. And I have tried to stay humble, yet I don't have to try hard: Both of them are quick to tell me if they disagree with me or if they question me. I take that as a good thing, because it means they feel like they can communicate freely with me, like equals, and that they haven't shut me out. …

I have a long way to go in learning how to teach, and in fact, I don't think you can ever become a "perfect teacher," because there's always more to learn. Still, I think I've improved, and I'm on a better path than the one on which I started. As I poise myself to dive into the pool of being a clinical instructor next year, I must admit, the diving board feels quite wobbly beneath me. What if I slip? Or what if I put too much or too little effort into my approach?

Or, recalling my memories from first grade, what if I lose my focus and do a back-flop? What if all this practice does not, in the end, prepare me for the big event? Well, I may not ever be Greg Louganis, and I may end up with a sore back, but I'm willing to get my feet—and legs, and chest, and hair—soaking wet.

REFLECTIONS FOR NEW NURSE EDUCATORS

Most studies of role transition in the workplace have focused on students transitioning to new nurse graduate positions or staff nurses transitioning to practitioner positions. There has been little research focused on the transition from clinician to nurse educator (Duffy, 2013; Spencer, 2013). Studies have pointed out that nurse clinicians who leave the security of their clinical position to assume a nurse educator role often describe their experience as stressful, frightening, and overwhelming, with feelings of apprehension, ambivalence, and uncertainty about their career move (Spencer, 2013, Weidman, 2013). It was clear from interviews with participants in this study, however, that clinicians also approach this transition with excitement and a genuine desire to share their knowledge with others.

A New Paradigm

Benner (2001) noted that expert clinical nurses find it difficult to address a problem by breaking it down, step by step, in a specific situation because they have accumulated experience that allows them to act intuitively, without having to rely on rubrics or rules to formulate answers to clinical problems. Yet, when thrust back into the novice role again, this step-by-step approach is exactly what is required for the novice to make the transition. Thus, this requires the expert to make a paradigm shift in the relearning of new information as a novice and leads to stress and frustration (Weidman, 2013). Weidman found that when she asked clinicians in her study why they decided to transition to nurse educators, they overwhelmingly responded that they wanted to share their expert knowledge through teaching. Thus, as suggested by participants in the study described here, expert clinicians may know *what* they should teach, but need help in knowing *how* to teach (Spencer, 2013).

Preparation for Transitioning to the Novice Nurse Educator Role

Estelle shared this reflection after attending some of the sessions of the Clinical Nurse Educator Academy:

> It is a very challenging journey for the new nurse educa-tor to become a novice again. … It would be a good idea to develop a pathway for the novice faculty and it should include all the skills needed to be successful faculty and how to achieve those skills. The checklist should also include different levels according to individual pace, personality, culture, and learning style.
>
> In the service area or hospital where new graduates are hired, they get at least 3 weeks of theory and 3 months of practice with a preceptor one on one. Why should it be dif-ferent for a new educator who is also new to the field? Are we preparing our educators to be successful in their field? Are we providing enough support and enabling environ-ment? … I strongly felt when new faculty talked yesterday about their new career as educators they definitely looked overwhelmed and overworked. If an expert clinician wanted to be an educator in her 40s, she doesn't want to change her career and then fail. … The question is: What kind of mentoring are we providing?

Naomi had been a clinical educator for a short time previously, but had enrolled in the academy to learn more about teaching. Her story also reflects the lack of preparation she received for this role:

> My first experience as a clinical educator was many years ago. My qualifications for this job were clinical experience and a willingness to work with students. There was no formal education or orientation offered for my new respon-sibilities. Not knowing what I should know about clinical

education was a bit like playing pin the tail on the donkey. I realize now that I didn't know enough to ask meaningful questions. I was in my own world. The nursing school provided me with a copy of course objectives, the student textbook was available, and a copy of the labs the students had completed.

I remember being so excited about beginning my new role in clinical teaching; I wanted to share everything I knew. These students were also enthusiastic about being in the clinical setting. They were like little sponges absorbing as much as they could, or at least most of the students were like this. It is mentally challenging and exhausting trying to find ways to engage these other students. Now I realize my teaching style may have been the problem.... Had I known then what I know now, I might have possibly stayed in that teaching arena.... A workshop such as the Nurse Educator Academy that covers specific topics would have been a dream come true. I didn't realize how much I didn't know about what I was doing until I'd been in the role for several years.

It is clear from Estelle, Naomi, and other research participants, as well as the literature, that clinicians often receive very little formal training in how to teach in their new role as clinical nurse educators (Duffy, 2013). Researchers in one study of 75 clinical nurse educators found that 31% of the educators had received no training at all for their new role (Suplee, Gardner, & Jerome-D'Emilia, 2014). Clinicians hired as part-time clinical nurse educators in their own institution may not even have opportunities to work alongside full-time faculty, who could help to mentor them in the challenges they are likely to face in clinical teaching (Spencer, 2013).

Poindexter (2013) noted that competencies associated with expert nurse educator practice have been identified, but expectations for entry-level competencies have not been clearly identified. Thus, Poindexter implemented a national survey ($n = 374$) to identify administrators' perceptions of expected competencies of entry-level novice educators for a full-time teaching position in the nursing program. Although the survey focused on full-time teaching positions so findings may not be generalizable to novice faculty who are assuming part-time clinical educator positions, it is interesting that the perceived competencies varied according to the mission of the institution. Although expectations for novice educators in nontenure positions focused on teaching and practice, expectations from research-intensive institutions placed high value on conducting research and emphasizing scholar role competencies. Thus, for part-time clinical faculty in research-intensive institutions, it would be important to clarify how expectations for these faculty differ from those of full-time positions.

Novice nurse educators are expected to assume entry-level teaching positions with specific levels of established competencies, but it is not clear how they will gain these competencies, given that preparation for their role is so limited. In Poindexter's (2013) study, competency related to leadership was consistently ranked high in expected levels of performance across all types of institutions. This raises questions for school of nursing or hospital personnel who are recruiting nurse clinicians for faculty roles. In addition to nursing practice skills and assuming the role of a novice nurse educator, is it realistic to expect leadership and scholarship competencies? How do novice nurse educators obtain the guidance needed to develop appropriate competences that are deemed important in an academic environment?

A variety of models are described in the literature for orienting and preparing expert nurse clinicians for the nurse educator role, but there is little consensus in the literature to support a single approach (Flood & Powers, 2012; Gilbert & Womack, 2012; Reid, Hinderer, Jarosinski, Mister, & Seldomridge, 2013). Feedback from the Clinical Nurse Educator Academy described here confirmed that structured information sessions were helpful, but the most important element was the opportunity for participants to share stories with each other about their background, goals, and fears in moving into a novice nurse educator role. Most of them had been so busy in their own clinical roles that they had not experienced opportunities to share ideas with each other. In the busy context of education and health care today, it is difficult to plan and implement extensive preparation programs for new nurse educators, but it is important to provide simple opportunities for them to share stories of goals, fears, successes, and failures. There is a need for more research on the experiences of clinicians in transitioning to the role of the nurse educator so that we can better prepare nurses for this important role.

Strategies for Successful Transition to the Novice Nurse Educator Role

- Identify your reasons for deciding to transition to the educator role so that you will know what you hope to gain from the experience.
- Identify the strengths that you bring to the educator role, as well as areas where you believe you need more guidance.
- Share your ideas and concerns with others in the nurse educator role.
- Find a mentor whose advice you trust.
- Keep a journal that describes your experiences so that you can judge your progress and competence in your new role.

Questions for Reflection

1. A colleague tells you that she has decided to pursue an adjunct nurse educator position in order to advance her position on her clinical career ladder. How would you respond?
2. A friend in your hospital has been asked to be a preceptor for a new graduate. She is a fairly new graduate herself and is unsure if she can be an effective preceptor. What advice would you give her?
3. Do you think the competencies for part-time nurse educators should be the same as those for full-time nurse educators?
4. What do you think are the most essential competencies for novice nurse educators to bring to their new role?
5. What do you think are the most common areas of preparation that novice nurse educators need?

REFERENCES

American Association of Colleges of Nursing. (2014). *Nursing faculty shortage.* Retrieved August 18, 2014, from www.aacn.nche.edu/media-relations/fact-sheets/nursing-faculty-shortage

Anderson, J. K. (2009). The work-role transition of expert clinicians to novice academic educator. *Journal of Nursing Education, 48,* 203–208.

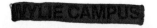

Benner, P. (1982). From novice to expert. *American Journal of Nursing, 82*(3), 402–407.

Benner, P. (2001). *From novice to expert: Excellence and power in clinical nursing practice* (Rev. ed.). Upper Saddle River, NJ: Prentice Hall.

Cangelosi, P. R., Crocker, S., & Sorrell, J. M. (2009). Expert to novice: Clinicians learning new roles as clinical nurse educators. *Nursing Education Perspectives, 30*, 367–371.

Culleiton, A. L., & Shellenbarger, T. (2007). Transition of a bedside clinician to a nurse educator. *MEDSURG Nursing, 16*, 253–257.

Duffy, R. (2013). Nurse to educator? Academic roles and the formation of personal academic identities. *Nurse Education Today, 33*, 620–624.

Flood, L. S., & Powers, M. E. (2012). Lessons learned from an accelerated post-master's nurse educator certificate program: Teaching the practicum course. *Nursing Education Perspectives, 33*(1), 40–44.

Gilbert, C., & Womack, B. (2012). Successful transition from expert nurse to novice nurse educator? Expert educator: It's about you! *Teaching and Learning in Nursing, 7*, 100–102.

Nurse Executive Center. (2008). *Bridging the preparation-practice gap. Volume I: Quantifying new graduate nurse improvement needs.* Washington, DC: The Advisory Board Company.

Poindexter, K. (2013). Novice nurse educator entry-level competency to teach: A national study. *Journal of Nursing Education, 52*(10), 559–566.

Reid, T. P., Hinderer, K. A., Jarosinski, J. M., Mister, B. J., & Seldomridge, L. A. (2013). Expert clinician to clinical teacher: Developing a faculty academy and mentoring initiative. *Nurse Education in Practice, 13*, 288–293.

Robert Wood Johnson Foundation. (2014). Nursing job outlook sunny as experts project need for more than one million new nurses by 2022. Retrieved from www.rwjf.org/en/about-rwjf/newsroom/newsroom-content/2014/05/long-term-job-outlook-for-nurses-is-sunny--as-experts-project-na.html

Schriner, C. L. (2007). The influence of culture on clinical nurses transitioning into the faculty role. *Nursing Education Perspectives, 28*, 145–149.

Spencer, C. (2013). From bedside to classroom: From expert back to novice. *Teaching and Learning in Nursing, 8*, 13–16.

Suplee, P. D., Gardner, M., & Jerome-D'Emilia, B. (2014). Nursing faculty preparedness for clinical teaching. *Journal of Nursing Education, 53*(3, Suppl.), S38–S41.

Weidman, N. A. (2013). The lived experience of the transition of the clinical nurse expert to the novice nurse educator. *Teaching and Learning in Nursing, 8*, 102–109.

Chapter 2

Making a Difference

Simply offering a harrowed family member a cup of coffee may make a difference. Sitting patiently as they express their fears or ask questions means so much.

—Fiona

Many nurses have voiced that they entered nursing because they "want to make a difference" in the lives of their future patients. Some of these nurses had personal experiences with nurses or the health care field in general that fueled this desire, while some "felt a calling" to do this. Regardless of the reasons why one became a nurse, often the passion for "making a difference" surfaces both in one's conversations and actions.

Moving to a nurse educator role allows a nurse to make a difference not only for patients and families, but also for students. The transition, however, may be difficult. One nurse educator described her concerns in leaving her clinician role for the new role of a nurse educator:

> I struggled with concerns about what I might miss, not
> so much when I was adjunct faculty and working as both
> a clinician and an educator, but when I went to full-time

teaching. I loved clinical and the close contact with patients and it was really hard for me to give up that kind of relationship. When I worked with students in the clinical area, the patients were not "mine" in the same way. I still had responsibility for them but it was different. I finally convinced myself that my students were "my patients" and I would make an important difference that way by helping them learn to take care of patients.

THE STORIES

Expert clinical nurses frequently have positive experiences precepting nursing students. From this involvement, many elect to become clinical instructors for nursing students in addition to their rigorous full-time clinical positions. These expert clinicians stated that they "want to share my knowledge with future nurses" and "make a difference in the education of our future." Their state-of-the-art mastery of clinical skills and health care practices are valuable models and resources for students. This chapter presents stories from the Cangelosi, Crocker, and Sorrell (2009) study centered on research participants' responses to the following prompt:

> Think about how you feel you make a difference for your patients as a clinician. Describe an incident that reflects your ideas about how you can make a difference for students as they learn new clinical skills.

Fiona's response presented at the start of this chapter reveals that even the most basic activities can make a real difference for a patient's family. It also uncovers the ripple effect of this "making a difference" passion. The ripple effect occurs when the care originally intended for one entity, such as the family, unintentionally extends to the patient, and even to the student caring for the patient. Although high-tech care and expert clinical knowledge are vital for "making a difference," little gestures and acts of kindness are also critically important. The reflections to this prompt clearly disclosed that patients, family members, and students benefited from these "making a difference" acts, making the ripple effect very evident.

Making a Difference for Patients and Their Families

It was clear from participants' responses that even as nurse educators, they wanted to continue to make a difference for patients and their families. Joanie described how "making a difference" may not be what one first may think. For her, visible and tangible signs of caring constitute "making a difference":

> Although my patients (sick neonates) could not verbalize to me that I made a difference, I have received comments and cards from their parents who felt positively affected by my care. Interestingly, however, there were never any remarks about how proficiently I hung the IV drips, or managed the infant on the ventilator, or how I accurately interpreted their child's lab results. Granted, these are important and necessary skills to possess, but these are not what the parents identify as making a difference. What parents remembered and articulated were instances of caring behavior that [were] perceived as genuine, honest, and open (e.g., staying long past shift change to support and talk to the parents, asking about their other children, acknowledging personal sorrow when the outcome is not good, or just being friendly and positive).

Callie revealed that in the psychiatric setting, "making a difference" may be as simple and as difficult as believing in the patient:

> I am currently working with a young male patient, whom I will give the pseudonym Brian. Brian suffers from a multitude of psychiatric diagnoses, which include bipolar disorder, borderline personality disorder, attention deficit disorder, and he is addicted to crack cocaine. He was admitted to the unit after cutting his wrists with a broken crack pipe in an attempt to kill himself. At only 22, he has been in and out of psychiatric treatment and drug rehab since age 13. Even for the most experienced and empathetic PMH [psychiatric mental health] nurse, this presentation, history, and combination of diagnoses could equate to an inability to succeed in treatment. I met Brian 2 days after

his admission and worked hard to establish a trusting rapport—the first intervention a PMH nurse must use if one expects any further interventions to be successful.

Although Brian would easily talk to me, it took several days for him to trust me and for me to trust him. Throughout the course of his admission, he had several episodes of yelling and screaming, refusing to participate in group therapy sessions, extreme mood lability, and high levels of anxiety. He required much time from the nurses, either seeking reassurance, medications, or preventing crises.

As Brian and I worked together, he allowed me into his world—a young life emotionally abandoned from childhood with no feelings of belonging or self-worth. He continued a life of drug addiction because he felt that was all people ever thought he would be. Even though he wanted to think otherwise, he had been written off for years by family and treatment providers as nothing more than an emotionally unstable crack addict. In listening to report and team rounds, I found that members of our own team felt the same way—they figured that Brian's history and difficulty aligning in treatment meant he was unmotivated and manipulative. Even though I appreciated Brian's potential ability to manipulate situations (he admitted he had done so in the past) and was not sure if he had the maturity to be able to handle the intense emotional crises he was currently experiencing, I knew it was my job to believe in him. If I, as a PMH nurse, could not believe he could succeed in treatment, then he would never believe it himself, and he never would succeed.

He is now preparing for discharge to a long-term dual diagnosis treatment facility, and although fearful and apprehensive, he now smiles when I give him positive feedback and acknowledges his progress in treatment thus far. He has practiced doing things he does not want to do, like go to AA [Alcoholics Anonymous] meetings, and has practiced regulating his own mood lability through artwork, music, and anxiety-reduction techniques. He is beginning to learn the skills needed to manage his bevy of psychiatric diagnoses. Even though I cannot guarantee he will indeed succeed in

treatment, I hope that my influence will help him whenever
that time comes. I feel I have done the very best job
I could have done as Brian's nurse simply because I believed
in him. I hope I have made a difference in his life.

Donna, similar to Fiona, shared that the little kindnesses shown to
patients can make the difference:

My patient was 32 weeks pregnant with an abruption that
resulted in IUFD [intrauterine fetal demise], excessive ante-
partum hemorrhage, and DIC [disseminated intravascular
coagulation]. Many professionals with different areas of
expertise were present and were helping to manage the
patient. She called me closer and told me how she felt so
thirsty and dehydrated. I gave her ice chips, which made
all the difference. She thanked me so much and verbalized
to me how she felt and the only big thing she remembered
was eating the ice chips. It was joyful to watch a smile on
her face. I made the difference.

Anne also worked on a psychiatric unit. For her, "making a difference" for her patient and the patient's family was similar to becoming a
novice again, because it required her to step out of her "comfort zone":

One of these incidents happened about 4 years ago. I was
working as an evening charge nurse on a research child
psychiatry unit. A 10-year-old boy was admitted to our unit
for observation of child-onset schizophrenia. The family was
from Vermont. They were very liberal, did not like rules,
and were heavily involved in an alternative lifestyle. Well, a
family that doesn't like and disregards rules on a psych unit
is bad news for anyone. The staff could not stand the family.
The father was the worst. He would get his son from the din-
ner table, turn him around in the same chair and then turn
on the television—even though there were other children
still eating and staff was right there. Every evening he would
come in and test some limit. He would wait for the staff to
react and then roll his eyes, blow out of his mouth, and make
a snide remark about how unintellectual the staff was. I have

to say—he was by far one of my least favorite people. Every time the door buzzer would go off and I saw him on the other side of the door, I could feel my mind and body chemically react to his presence. But, I was the charge nurse and was determined not to let him affect me professionally.

Well, one evening, the father was on the unit and the usual scenario played out. The father tested a limit on the rules and the nurse needed to address the situation—nothing new. But, out of the corner of my eye, I saw the father heading—or shall I say "storming"—out the door. I knew there was something wrong. The easiest thing to do was to let him go and enjoy the rest of my evening. Although I could not stand the guy, I knew I had to do something. I ran to the end of the hall and met him in the threshold of the entrance to the unit right before the door was closing. I said, "Mr. Smith—you don't look happy. What happened?" Initially, he looked completely shocked—shocked that anyone actually cared about how he was feeling. After about a 10-second silence, he told me that he didn't like the nurse working with his son, she was too harsh and she was chewing gum (Nicorette) and it was just making him angry. He just started flooding. I told him that I understood how he feels and that actually the whole staff understands the tremendous sorrow and heartache he has every day when he sees his son and knows that he will never have a normal life. I assured him that we did not see his son as a patient, but as an adorable kid with a sweet and quirky sense of humor who is here helping us out with our research. After our little chat, there was a brief smile from him. His son was with us for 6 additional months. His father never had a problem with the staff or the unit rules after our talk. In fact, he was quite pleasant.

This incident has stayed with me. It's because I faced one of my fears—confrontation—and went forward and dove in and addressed the problem (even when there was an easy way out). The outcome was the best possible—a content parent and a happy staff. I also learned a valuable lesson: Do not assume that the patient on the unit is the only one who needs care. Yes, I know—we learned about caring for the whole family in nursing school, blah, blah, blah…. But, this gentleman was in his mid-30s, in good physical health, and gainfully employed—not patient or "I need help" material. Unfortunately, his behaviors were so unappealing that the staff just distanced themselves from him because he caused so much angst on the unit. What really needed to happen was for the staff to get closer to him and not distance themselves from someone who initially came across as "difficult." But how was I ever going to experience this success first-hand if I didn't leave my introverted world of pleasantness? People do not want to step out of their comfort zone. But, I made such a difference stepping out of my comfort zone…it is important to not get too comfortable or you may miss something—like I did with Mr. Smith. This is why I remember this incident very clearly. It was one of my shining moments.

Making a Difference for Nursing Students

Joanie described how the clinical experiences she valued also related to her new educator role:

The same principles are applicable in the educational setting as we "care for" our nursing students. … Recently, I had a very distressing phone conversation with the mother of a nursing student. I was calling the student to confirm her position as a nurse extern for the upcoming summer. The student's mother answered the phone, stated that her daughter was not home and asked if she could give her daughter a message. I explained that I wanted to see if her daughter had any questions or concerns about her new job, to discuss her orientation, schedule, and shift preferences. The mother paused and asked if she could briefly talk with me. (In retrospect, I think that I was caught off guard and didn't even consider that her daughter might not approve of this conversation, as I replied "sure.") This mother sounded tearful and very anxious as she started to speak. The mother stated that she was a

nurse in the same hospital that her daughter did her clinical rotations, and sadly admitted that her daughter did not
have good experiences. The nurses were not welcoming,
the atmosphere was hostile, and her daughter was miser-
able. She pleaded with me to place her daughter on any
shift, as long as her preceptor was "nice."

I was embarrassed that this mother had to even make
such a request. After expressing my concerns for this student, I did offer a few suggestions. First, I encouraged her to
have her daughter speak to her clinical instructors, as they
are the students' advocates and advisors. Hopefully, the
clinical instructors would apprise the unit managers of any
issues. Second, I said that I would *not* advise her daughter
to "grow thicker skin," as that just takes away from our gentle, caring nature, but rather to learn from these situations.
I encouraged this mother to tell her daughter what I tell
new graduate nurses: "Although there is much for new
nurses to learn, new nurses have so much to teach us all
about being excited, energetic, positive, and open to new
experiences. New nurses need to feel empowered to model
good behavior and not to tolerate negative conduct." This
mother did not speak to the skills that her daughter did or
did not gain during these clinical experiences. What broke
this mother's heart was the way her daughter was treated
by the very people who make up her chosen profession.

It is clear that Joanie will continue to make a difference for patients and
families, but may have even more influence by caring for her students.

An "advocacy gene" is what Fiona feels enables her to make a
difference with nursing students. Perhaps this is true. However, it is
amazing how even minimal help with routine tasks, patience, and—
again—belief in someone can make such a difference:

I believe that my advocacy gene has accompanied me from
my former role as a clinician to my current role as an educator. Remembering that students are people too is something I hope I never forget. One incident that reflects how I
think I make a difference in my students' performances as
they learn new clinical skills happened just recently. One

of my students had an order to insert a nasogastric tube in her patient. When she came to me with the order, she was terrified. "I have only done this in the lab on a dummy. I'm really not sure I can do this." I took the student to a quiet area of the unit and explained to her that I had been with her in lab and had seen her excellent technique. I was sure that she could do this and told her so, but also let her know that I would be right beside her all the way. We gathered the supplies and returned to the quiet area. I asked her to take a deep breath and tell me everything she could about the procedure. She was able to list all of the steps correctly and had all of the right answers to my questions.

When we entered the room, she was amazing. I don't think I have ever performed this procedure as smoothly as she did. After leaving the room, I told her exactly that. Her response was, "I was able to do it because you were so patient with me and I didn't want to let you down." She thanked me for having such confidence in her and I could see on her face that she felt very proud of her accomplishment. I believe that if I can maintain this attitude and let the students know that, "Yes, you can," I will make a difference.

Sabrina noted how the realistic simulation she created for nursing care at the end of life has made a difference for her students. Although the simulation indeed has an impact, it is the caring manner in which Sabrina deals with the impact that is most revealing:

One example of how I have made a difference to students is what has happened during the end of life (eol) simulation that I do with students. One student in particular realized after going through the simulation that she really had some issues with grief, and I helped her to access a grief support group through the organization I work for. The simulation I created is very authentic and has proven to be very powerful for some students in terms of tapping into their own histories with death and dying. I try to be very honest and very gentle with the students during the simulation, and I've come to understand that what helps them the most is the understanding and "detoxifying," if you

will, of the whole dying process. Of course it's *essential* to
do this in a gentle and caring way, because the topic can be
so scary and emotionally charged.

Lisa disclosed how the development of a password with her RN to BSN
student made the difference in helping him gain confidence in the clinical
setting. Through this simple password or question, Lisa assisted this student in becoming more self-assured in a very caring and dignified manner:

> On his first day on the unit, he was introduced to all the
> staff, the PCD [patient care director], and the environment.
> He observed me throughout the shift and I provided him
> with time to become familiar with the computer documen-
> tation. I observed him becoming eager to learn. The next
> day I assigned him two patients and observed him com-
> plete his assessment on the first patient. We then retreated
> to the nursing station for feedback. He proceeded with
> the next patient, however, when something was missed or
> skipped, we had a code for me to step in and assist him.
> I would ask, "May I help you with …?" to which the stu-
> dent would reply, "Thank you." By the third week, I added
> another patient to his group and would seek out patients
> requiring procedures such as Corpak tube placement, any
> type of wound care, tracheostomy care, lumbar drain,
> Jackson-Pratt drain, and chest tubes so that he could prac-
> tice and, for this, he was grateful.
>
> By mid-semester, this student was gaining self-
> confidence in his skills. All I had to do was to discuss
> procedure steps with him. He would collect the correct
> supplies, confirm them with me, and he would then com-
> plete the procedure without difficulty. He became familiar
> with the routine on the unit, such as discharge rounds
> on Wednesdays. He participated in these rounds, which
> means he had knowledge of a patient's medical condition
> as well as social/family issues.
>
> By the end of spring, this student was more like a regu-
> lar nurse on the unit and other nurses were asking for his
> assistance. He finally had the confidence needed to practice
> his skills.

Marian described her passion for making a difference for students in the psychiatric specialty that she loved:

> We have all established that education is an ongoing learning process and we as nurse educators have a responsibility to provide our students with all the necessary tools possible so that adequate learning takes place. So what does this mean? As a seasoned nurse with many years of experience, I take time to talk with all of the student nurse groups that come to psychiatry. My focus is to alleviate any fears they may have and welcome them in a comfortable, accepting manner. I share the different types of patients we treat and tell mini stories to prepare them for their experiences. I discuss the good and the bad.
>
> Developing a relationship with your student nurses is important. They need to be accepted. Often they walk into cold and hostile ground. I provide them with warmth, nurturing, and an open door. I explain to them that we all have been in their shoes. I let them know it is ok to be apprehensive.... And when it is all over and done, these students who started out scared and naïve leave with confidence and acceptance. Accepting of a specialty that has been so tainted by others because we as humans are in denial about psychiatry. Mainly because we do not confront our own issues because it's too painful.... Those of us who enjoy psychiatry have a duty to share the specialty in a way that it is respected and understood. As a clinical specialist in this area, I have a duty to explain the behaviors and help others understand. This is how I make a difference. Taking time and sharing. Taking time and explaining. Alleviating fears and instilling confidence.... Finally, this is how I make a difference, by just being me and giving of myself.

Making a Difference for Patients, Families, and Nursing Students

Many of the participants quickly realized the ripple effect of "making a difference" when they recalled incidents where both patients and nursing students were affected. Although these incidents may seem routine in a nurse's day, the sensitivity or tact (discussed further in Chapter 3) in how the patients, families, and students were approached had a profound, positive, and lasting influence on all involved, including the participants who recounted these occurrences. For these participants, the incidents reinforced why they wanted to become novices again and learn how to move from an expert clinician and preceptor to an expert clinical instructor. Eileen shared this story:

> I had the opportunity to precept a student in her senior year, and with her assistance, to streamline a teaching/ learning strategy. Using the school's preceptor workbook and the student's syllabus as a framework, a 6-week schedule of objectives was agreed upon. A contract was worked out to clarify student and preceptor responsibilities, and a timeline for accomplishing objectives was established.
>
> Four weeks into the clinical rotation the student was exhibiting professional behaviors and was completing assessments and patient care on three mother–baby couples, with the appropriate level of competence and autonomy as outlined in the syllabus. It was about this time that a patient came into our lives that afforded an opportunity for the student to manage a patient with rapidly changing acuity.
>
> Together we admitted a patient that was 2 hours postpartum from an emergency cesarean section surgery. The mother was stable on admission, and we received a report from the labor and delivery nurse that was unremarkable for history. Her husband and mother were at the bedside. The student was familiar with the standard of care for a C-section patient. After obtaining the first set of vital signs, the student made notes as I relayed information about my hands-on assessment. The patient had been with us 1 hour when the second assessment was due.
>
> As we entered the patient room for the second assessment, there was a noticeable difference in our patient. She was clammy and pale, had a normal respiration rate and temperature, but had an increased heart rate (HR 140). The blood pressure was 100/60. After making a preliminary assessment and ruling out a postpartum hemorrhage,

a nasal cannula with 3 L of oxygen was placed on the patient. I asked the student to gather supplies for starting an IV. Then, I started making phone call: first to the doctor, and then to my charge nurse. I had a feeling I was looking at either a postpartum hemorrhage or possible pulmonary embolism. I remained at the bedside and waited for the obstetrician to arrive.

Within minutes, the doctor was at the bedside evaluating the situation and ordering labs and x-rays. At one point, we had the nurse manager, the charge nurse, the doctor, and a nurse's aide in the room with us, offering assistance. Everyone was professional, attentive, and reassuring to both the patient and her husband and mother. The student was also comforting to the family. The patient was eventually transferred to the intensive care unit with a falling blood pressure and tachycardia.

While we were involved with our acute patient, the charge nurse assumed responsibility for the other two mother–baby couples assigned to us. After documenting the transfer, a short debrief was made. The student recalled how smoothly the collaboration and communication went, and how following the nursing process assisted the doctor in making a diagnosis and treatment plan. This made the student feel secure that in a similar situation, she would be supported by her colleagues. I made sure I commended her on her professionalism and her efforts to comfort the family.

Although we had this patient for a short time, I believe we made a difference to the patient and her family, in keeping them updated and informed, while making sure every resource was followed up that related to her care. The patient's family sought us out after the patient was transferred, to thank us for supporting them and keeping them informed. Again, this was a unique opportunity to mentor a student through a stressful situation, and watch her grow as a nurse, and make a difference in her journey.

Olivia described how her calm demeanor and consideration for both the patient and the new graduate nurse made a positive difference for all involved. She also shared how experiences such as this give her "inner reward and fulfillment as a clinician," which, not surprisingly, is what she is beginning to experience as a novice clinical educator as well:

> I had a patient about 1 year ago who developed complications after she delivered her baby. The nurse that gave me report said that Mrs. D was very sick and very needy. The patient was 48 hours post-cesarean section with symptoms of abdominal distension, nausea, and vomiting. She had her nasogastric [NG] tube to low continuous suction and her diagnosis was postoperative ileus. Mrs. D was from India and spoke very little English. Her husband was very fluent in English.... After taking report on Mrs. D, I explained Mrs. D's condition, diagnosis, and the plan of care to new graduate RN, Linda, who I was precepting. Linda was anxious, because this would be the first postoperative ileus patient she would care for. I reassured Linda that I will do everything possible to make this a good learning experience for her, and that she should not hesitate to stop and ask me any question about Mrs. D. I went to the room to check on the patient and to let her know that I would be her night nurse and that I would be working with Linda, a new graduate nurse. When Linda and I went into the room to assess the patient, Mrs. D looked very uncomfortable. The patient said she was in pain and identified her pain level to be between seven and eight on a ten scale. Mrs. D was medicated with Demerol 50 mg and Vistaril 25 mg IV by Linda. At this point, Linda was feeling comfortable with caring for Mrs. D. I asked Linda how comfortable she was with flushing the NG tube, and she said that this was her first time. I reassured her and gave her instructions according to the hospital's policy and procedure on how to check placement and how to flush an NG tube. After checking placement, Linda flushed and the NG tube started draining. Mrs. D felt an immediate relief and expressed her gratitude right there at the bedside. With

guidance and few instructions, Linda performed a head-to-toe assessment on the patient and also assessed her pain level. By this time, the patient was more relaxed, and her pain level went from eight to two, and her NG tube was draining without difficulty. Linda was able to assess Mrs. D's baby and assisted her in providing care for her baby as she had intravenous fluid running for the first 2 days. Mrs. D was NPO [nothing by mouth] for the first 48 hours. The next night I still had Linda with me and she was able to see the improvement in Mrs. D's condition. The patient and her husband were very pleased with the care she received and expressed their gratitude about the special care given during her hospital stay. The excellent care given to Mrs. D made a difference in her recovery, and the guidance Linda received made her feel competent in her ability to care for this complex patient.

REFLECTIONS FOR NEW NURSE EDUCATORS

These "making a difference" stories from expert clinicians/novice educators are what Taylor (2005) described as the "detailed explorations of people tangled in the messiness of living" (p. 11). Taylor further stated, "We love to hear stories because they are mostly about human beings surviving trouble" (p. 174). Stories also allow one to reflect and learn from experiences, as do the narratives included here. The expert clinicians in the Clinical Nurse Educator Academy openly shared how, upon reflection, they really felt they made a difference in the life of a patient, family, or student. The ripple effect was a byproduct of this, and was noted by the researchers only after analyzing the stories. Perhaps these stories do represent "just another day's work" in the life of a nurse, but they indeed reflect the powerful difference these nurses made for those they worked with. The narratives also reflect how these novice educators were already fulfilling the National League for Nursing (2005) first core competency for nurse educators: Facilitate learning.

The novice educators' stories involving nursing students mirror student comments as to what makes an effective clinical instructor. In a hermeneutic phenomenological study analyzing the experiences of 19 accelerated second-degree students, Cangelosi (2007) found that clinical instructors had the greatest impact on students' learning. Marsha, now a telemetry nurse, described a situation with her clinical instructor that made a real difference for her:

> I remember being in clinical one day, and the [patient] had a colostomy. And I remember looking at my clinical instructor, who had years of knowledge to build on, and looking at her and giving her that blank stare. And she took the 10 minutes necessary to say, "If it's here, it's this; if it's here, it's this; if it's this, it's this; and this is what you do." And that made the difference, so that now if I see a colostomy, I'm not so scared of it, and I ask people questions. Being exposed to it and having it explained to me on the spot—that made the difference, because we did not get the colostomy lecture until springtime. (Cangelosi, 2007, p. 402)

Marsha revealed that not only was the hands-on instruction so vital and so memorable, but the "pedagogical moment" (van Manen, 1991, p. 40), the teachable moment, or the just-in-time teaching, made such a difference, that to this day as a practicing nurse, she remembers and applies what this clinical instructor taught her. Both the accelerated students in this study and the novice educators in the academy described effective clinical instructors as able to see the "pedagogical possibilities in ordinary incidents" (van Manen, 1991, p. 187).

In another qualitative study with accelerated nursing students, Rico, Beal, and Davies (2010) noted that accelerated nursing students report learning best from clinical faculty who share their own patient experiences. In their study for the Carnegie Foundation for the Advancement of Teaching, Benner, Sutphen, Leonard, and Day (2010) also reported the teaching and learning effectiveness of faculty sharing with students their own clinical encounters with patients. Now, who is in a better position to do this than expert clinicians who want to teach nursing students? Not only would quality teaching be performed, but many positive experiences would also be made for the students, the instructors, and patients. With careful mentoring and instruction in the practice of teaching, expert clinicians can make a tremendous difference for students. As Callie astutely stated:

> Making a difference does not necessarily mean teaching the most complicated skills or giving the most challenging assignments. It means tailoring one's approach to meet the specific needs of each student while still meeting the expectations of the course. It means listening, empathizing, and giving each person a chance.... The vulnerable students who are just barely surviving can easily fall through the cracks and are written off by other educators. These are the students who disappear—just stop showing up to class one day or don't show up the next semester. As educators, we could have made a difference for these students, but we didn't, and now we have a few less future nurses.

Strategies for Making a Difference in Teaching Nursing Students

- Capitalize on the pedagogical moment.
- See the pedagogical possibilities in ordinary incidents.
- Share your own clinical experiences with students.
- Use a variety of teaching/learning strategies to accomplish the course objectives.
- Assign challenging patients, just be there to assist your student.
- Relate what the students are seeing in the clinical setting with what they are learning in the classroom. Know the curriculum in the school where you teach so you can do this.
- Do not be afraid to ask questions of the full-time faculty or clinical coordinator. They are to mentor you and assist you in learning about the school, teaching in academia, and the specific objectives of the course you are teaching. Keep their phone numbers/e-mail addresses handy.
- Listen to the students—what are they yearning to learn; what are they fearful of?
- Reflect on your teaching and clinical experiences—through reflection we learn.

Questions for Reflection

1. Think about your own nursing education. What made a difference for you?
2. Was there an instructor who made a difference for you? If so, in what way?
3. How have you made a difference for your patients? For families? For students?
4. What do you think is the most salient characteristic you have that will help you in teaching nursing students?
5. One of your clinical students is very fearful about performing any invasive procedure. How would you help this student learn to control her fear and function effectively in the clinical setting?
6. Do you think the concept of caring has a place in "making a difference," or do nurses just make a difference by the nature of the work they do?

REFERENCES

Benner, P., Sutphen, M., Leonard, V., & Day, L. (2010). *Educating nurses: A call for radical transformation.* San Francisco, CA: Jossey-Bass.

Cangelosi, P. R. (2007). Accelerated second-degree baccalaureate nursing programs: What is the significance of clinical instructors? *Journal of Nursing Education, 46,* 400–405.

Cangelosi, P. R., Crocker, S., & Sorrell, J. M. (2009). Expert to novice: Clinicians learning new roles as clinical nurse educators. *Nursing Education Perspectives, 30,* 367–371.

National League for Nursing. (2005). *Core competencies of nurse educators with task statements.* Retrieved from www.nln.org/profdev/corecompetencies.pdf

Rico, J. S., Beal, J., & Davies, T. (2010). Promising practices for faculty in accelerated nursing programs. *Journal of Nursing Education, 49,* 150–155.

Taylor, D. (2005). *Letters to my children. A father passes on his values.* St. Paul, MN: Bog Walk.

Van Manen, M. (1991). The tact of teaching. *The meaning of pedagogical thoughtfulness.* London, Ontario, Canada: Althouse.

CHAPTER 3

Power of Faculty: The Tact of Teaching

Staff made it clear that students were unwelcome by stating, "What? We have to have a student?! We don't even have anybody here that likes students!"

—Tanner-Garrett, 2014, p. 50

It is critical that nurse educators identify strategies to empower nursing students and new graduate nurses to implement caring behaviors in their own practice. In order for nurses to learn the importance of implementing caring behaviors with their patients and peers, it seems imperative that they see caring modeled for them in their educational experiences. Van Manen (1991) uses the term "tact" to describe a teaching approach that embodies thoughtful, mindful, caring interactions between faculty and students. Van Manen (1991) envisions tact as the space between theory and practice, noting that this tactful teaching can help us overcome the problem of separation between these two concepts. The tact of teaching is an important concept for new clinical nurse educators to address in order to help students apply theoretical knowledge in a learning context that values them as individuals.

THE STORIES

This chapter presents findings from three qualitative research studies that collected stories of undergraduate nursing students' experiences in the clinical setting. Nurse educators, as they struggle with day-to-day conflicts in implementing their role, often feel that they do not have a great deal of power. The stories here, however, illustrate that faculty, through their approach to connecting with students, have a great deal of power to create a caring learning environment. Stories of caring and uncaring experiences with faculty are presented first, followed by stories focused on how cultural factors and incivility may affect student learning in the clinical setting.

Stories of Caring and Uncaring

Twenty-one undergraduate students participated in a phenomenological study in which students described caring and uncaring incidents they had experienced in the clinical setting (Redmond & Sorrell, 1996; Sorrell & Redmond, 1997). As students in this study talked about experiences with their teachers, it was clear that faculty had a great deal of power and influence on the learning of their students—even though they may not have realized it.

Caring Behaviors. One student, Joan, described an incident when she needed to talk about a crisis she had with her patient and how helpful the faculty member was in providing an opportunity for her to do this:

> When I went on that morning I could tell that she [patient] was badly off. Later in the day, it became clear that she was dying and I sat with her as she died. I was having a hard time—I really didn't want to talk about it that day. The next morning my instructor told me that she really wanted to talk with me because she was really worried about what I was going through. She pulled me aside and we talked. It helped, it really did. We cried—it would still be bottled up inside of me if I hadn't talked to her about it. (Redmond & Sorrell, 1996, p. 23)

Joan talked about how moved she was that her instructor cried with her. It made her feel that it was okay to have these feelings of extreme sadness after watching her patient die. It also helped her to see that even as a student, she had been instrumental in helping to provide comfort and calm in her patient's last hours.

Another student, Carrie, reflected on an experience that happened many years earlier on her first day in the clinical area. She had been assigned to care for a young woman in the ICU who had leukemia. The patient suddenly began bleeding and died that day. No one explained to Carrie what had happened to cause her patient to die. Carrie described her feelings, "I remember thinking, feeling like I was floating, what did I not see?" Fortunately, the next day one of the nurses from the ICU made a special effort to seek out Carrie, who was then on a different unit. This nurse talked with Carrie about possible feelings of guilt that she sensed Carrie might have. She explained to Carrie, "You couldn't have done anything. Nobody knew that it would happen." As Carrie shared her story, the tears streamed down her face. Even though the incident had happened years earlier, it was clear that for her, the memory of that day was still very fresh:

> She sought me out, knowing that I would be somewhere
> in the hospital…and said, "I wanted to find you; are you
> okay?" And I thought, "Wow, that's caring, that's caring."
> It made a big difference. (Sorrell & Redmond, 1997, p. 231)

If this nurse had not gone out of her way to ensure that a student nurse knew that she was not to blame for her patient's death, Carrie may still be wondering whether she had caused harm to her patient.

Sharon described a simple incident that might have seemed insignificant to the faculty member but made a big impact on the class of stressed nursing students:

> I had an instructor stand up in front of the class and
> tell us in the middle of our junior year, when everybody
> was stressed out beyond belief, and everybody went
> home and cried every night: "I'm really sensing that you
> are all really frustrated. If you want to talk before you do
> something drastic, come to my office. I have tissues,

> I have candy, and we'll talk. But don't make any deci-
> sions without us." I wish more faculty could be like that,
> supportive instead of judgmental or so caught up in
> grading papers. (Redmond & Sorrell, 1996, p. 24)

Sharon's story illustrates the importance of anticipating students' needs in order to intervene appropriately. Her instructor monitored the nonverbal behavior of students in her class to identify the stress that they were experiencing. With the challenges teachers have preparing for classroom and clinical teaching, it is easy to forget that students are undergoing similar or even greater amounts of stress. Failing to identify this and intervene to reduce the stress may result in poor performance by the students or even their withdrawal from the program.

Nancy shared a humorous incident that illustrates the importance of faculty working together to help a student. She described how she naïvely dressed to attend a campus board of visitors meeting in her t-shirt and shorts, with her hair "all ratty looking." When the nursing dean explained that the meeting was formal, Nancy realized her error. Nevertheless, the dean went into action—she quickly gathered some faculty members to tell them of the problem and the faculty worked together to get Nancy prepared. They actually switched clothes with Nancy so that 15 minutes later she entered the board room with a professional (but undersized) suit, panty hose (barely reaching above her hemline), and nice pumps (almost two sizes too large). With hair now neatly combed and a blank piece of paper on which she pretended she had her speech, Nancy was ready for action. She said:

> I learned from that, the humor that had to remain in nurs-
> ing, and the caringness and cohesiveness of the faculty.
> They were just all so excited to see me fill the role. One
> of the faculty walked by and said, "That's what nurs-
> ing's all about. Just flexibility, working with whatever
> you have." The dean saw skills and things that she knew
> that I had that just really had been sheltered, laying there
> and hidden.... She saw in me so much potential and so
> she encouraged me into participating and promoting the
> nursing profession, and boy, have I! (Sorrell & Redmond,
> 1997, p. 231)

After graduation, Nancy made important contributions as a nurse in working with patients and students in developing countries. She obtained a master's and a PhD degree and is currently working as a nurse researcher and educator, implementing caring behaviors with her own students.

Uncaring Behaviors. Some of the "uncaring" stories that students shared were surprising to the researchers, who could see themselves unwittingly acting in similar ways with students. It is doubtful that the faculty members described in the following three stories realized the negative impact their actions had on the students.

Sarah, a beginning student with English as a second language (ESL), shared this story about the impact that a simple comment by her instructor had on her ability to think clearly and confidently:

> I told the professor I was unsure how to interpret an exam
> question. Her response was, "READ the question." Just the
> tone that she used to me, "Just READ the question," but I
> was interpreting it a couple of different ways, and I wanted
> clarification. I was very upset by that, VERY upset. It took me
> about 5 to 10 minutes to just sit there—and just calm down.
> (Redmond & Sorrell, 1996, p. 23)

Marie described the experience of giving her first injection to a patient. Probably every nurse remembers how difficult it was to "stick" a patient the first time, but with so many things to think about as a nurse educator, it is easy to forget the reassurance needed by students for this first injection. Marie described it this way:

> I thought I'd done a wonderful job. I gave an injection in
> front of another person to a patient who was in pain. In my
> postclinical conference, my teacher singled me out, out of
> nine other students, to tear apart my shot technique. She
> told me that I was wiggling and that I shouldn't have done
> that. I wobbled my hand a little bit. But, my patient said
> it was fine. I had to hurt another person to help them, and
> that's very stressful for me. I don't feel my teacher was there
> to give me support that I needed. There was a much better
> way that she could have confronted me with it, like, "There

is a different technique and next time we can work on it,"
or, "I'll show you how to hold your hand," as opposed to,
you know, in front of everybody, "You did it all wrong."
(Redmond & Sorrell, 1996, p. 23)

With the current shortage of full-time nurse educators, many schools are employing part-time faculty, especially for clinical teaching. The part-time faculty are often excellent clinicians and teachers but they are often somewhat isolated from the day-to-day course planning in which full-time faculty are engaged. Emily's story helps us see how important it is to include part-time or adjunct faculty in the planning of clinical teaching approaches. Emily described this experience:

Two instructors kind of played favorites. They would take
one group, the group they worked with, and go to lunch with
them, they went over to their house, and they exchanged
home visits and things. The other group (my group), which
was with the adjunct faculty, was excluded. You ended up
with a real division in the class and I think a lot of people felt
it. The more time you spent with the instructors, the more
you got to know them, you know what to expect of them.
(Redmond & Sorrell, 1996, p. 24)

Emily's comments point out that learning is not confined to the classroom or clinical setting. Gathering outside of the classroom where faculty and students share food or converse in a faculty member's home can provide opportunities for learning in a welcoming environment other than the classroom. It is important, however, that all students have equal opportunities to experience this.

Stories of Caring and Culture

Culture can be defined broadly as the attributes, language, physical characteristics, values, or behaviors that a group identifies as its own (Long, 2012). As the nursing profession becomes more diverse, it is critical that nurse educators consider how cultural issues may affect their students' learning. Students' stories from one study in an associate degree nursing program revealed how the insensitivity of faculty and others in the clinical environment can negatively affect learning (Glasgow, 2014). The research study focused on perceptions of faculty and students regarding factors that influence the communication and clinical skills of ESL nursing students. Using a qualitative case study design, the researcher interviewed five nursing faculty and entry-level ESL students to explore their perceptions of important supports and barriers to their learning. The researcher identified four themes that influenced the development of entry-level ESL nursing students' communication and clinical skills: (a) Lack of culturally sensitive teaching practices, (b) limited internal program cultural supports, (c) diverse cultural background barriers, and (d) insufficient cultural diversity training. One theme, lack of culturally sensitive teaching practices, is discussed here as an especially important consideration for the novice clinical nurse educator who is attempting to meet learning needs for a diverse student body.

Faculty participants in the study described their desire to create a culturally sensitive learning environment for their students but realized that cultural shortcomings existed within their teaching practices. One faculty member stated:

> Outside of our own cultures, there are so many things we do not know, and what we teach is based on our individual techniques.... We are told to promote cultural diversity and sensitivity with regard to patient care throughout all of the courses we teach, but in the case of cultural sensitivity toward students, there is no teaching standard to the curriculum.... Students become fearful of saying the wrong things, and in the clinical setting they are deterred from communicating with patients, which is necessary to practice nursing care skills. In clinical, these students are sometimes shown little patience and tolerance by patients. (Glasgow, 2014, p. 78)

Another faculty participant described her experiences with ESL students' nonverbal behaviors and attitudes:

> In clinical, I see a lot of ESL students who communicate with softer voices, show no eye contact, won't ask for help, and act a little more timid about touching, depending on what their culture is. Depending on their cultural background, an ESL student may have characteristics that

impede or give the impression that they do not understand. I can think of some [ESL students] in clinical I have
actually offended trying to communicate with them....
So, you have to find out if it's you [faculty] not explaining
things [well], or they [ESL students] are really not understanding for some reason. In clinical, all of these things can
make a big difference in ESL students' skills performances.
(Glasgow, 2014, p. 94)

Comments from student participants conveyed similar perceptions of
insensitive teaching practices they had experienced. One ESL student who
had lived in the United States and spoke English daily for 7 years stated:

Basically, our faculty looks at us like we are all even, so I
guess that could be viewed as supporting us.... I don't think
some of them take the time to get to know students' cultures,
which creates barriers for students from other cultures in this
program.... In clinical, I did experience one instructor who
tried to help me improve my communication and patient
care approach by telling me to not always voice everything
I am thinking, even though that is my culture. This faculty
told me that different cultures might perceive the meaning
of something different than from what was intended, which
is important when caring for patients in clinical. This helped
me in clinical by learning how to identify different words or
different ways of expressing communicating with patients
when performing my nursing skills. It helped me to interact
with patients and other people from different backgrounds,
which is important when I perform my nursing skills.
(Glasgow, 2014, p. 81)

Another student shared how her culture influenced interactions with
faculty:

Being of Asian culture, in the class, I don't talk to the professor. Sometimes, I envy American students when they
are talking to the professors, building relationships, and
joking with each other.... Some people think I am not competent about some things because I am so quiet, but that

is not true—it's just how my culture does things. If faculty just try to talk to me, smile, or just call my name, I would feel comfortable and it would help me to get involved and communicate more.... When faculty do engage with me, it builds my confidence level and I feel more comfortable talking to them and showing my skills in clinical. (Glasgow, 2014, pp. 96–97)

Some students in the study stated that they felt their cultural background contributed to faculty prejudging them. One student expressed this as follows:

I think that if faculty experienced ESL students' frustrations, they would understand where our frustrations come from and the cultural diversity challenges ESL students go through.... One personal experience I had was when my personal cultural accommodation was discussed openly in clinical in front of other students. This created embarrassment for me in the clinical area. This is why it would help to have open communication dialogue between students and faculty to learn about other cultures. Even though in my culture there are some things you just don't talk about with your friends or people from different cultures, learning about other cultures can prevent things like this from happening again. It also can impact how we interact with our patients, assess them, care for them. (Glasgow, 2014, p. 98)

The clinical setting creates significant challenges for culturally and linguistically diverse nursing students where language, cultural differences, and interpretation of cultural norms complicate the learning process (Harvey, Robinson, & Frohman, 2013). The cultural competence of nurse educators is essential for addressing these students' learning needs. Even experienced educators, however, may feel they lack the skills needed for effective cultural encounters in the clinical setting (Long, 2012).

Nurse educators need to acknowledge that they are in positions of power and should identify strategies for effectively addressing the needs of diverse students. Common teaching strategies for cultural competence include group discussion, lectures, case scenarios, simulation, clinical experiences, cultural immersion, and presentations by ethnic minority speakers (Long, 2012). Fitzsimmons (2009) suggests the use of experiential activities for nurse educators to help them understand the role of "the other" so that a trustful environment can be established that encourages questioning and self-expression (p. 97). She also suggests that faculty should implement open and honest discussions about racism so that all students feel more open in sharing feelings of discrimination that they have encountered in their educational experiences.

There has been limited research to evaluate the effectiveness of teaching interventions in cultural competence (Allen, Brown, Duff, Nesbitt, & Hepner, 2013; Davis, Davis, & Williams, 2010; Long, 2012). Findings of one study emphasized what Sarah's story reflected: that ESL students often need additional time to read and comprehend information (Crawford & Candlin, 2013). Implementing a program framed by a caring pedagogy, with the relationship between the student and teacher being highly interactive and connected, can help to foster dialogue, reflection, and trust—in essence, a caring relationship (Harvey et al., 2013). In the process, both faculty and students gain insight into their view of the world and new understandings of cross-cultural learning.

Civility in Nursing Education

One area in which nurse educators can make an important difference for their students is recognizing the possibility of incivility, or bullying, in their interactions with students and staff in the clinical environment. Tanner-Garrett (2014) used a case study approach to explore perceptions of eight new nurse graduates who described experiences of bullying that occurred while they were nursing students. The researcher described five themes that emerged from the face-to-face interviews: (a) bullying behaviors, (b) difficulty in defining bullying, (c) devaluation of students, (d) reduced learning, and (e) emotional responses to bullying.

Student participants described bullying as not just actions or words, but subtle behaviors such as eye-rolling, whispering behind someone's back, ignoring, and not speaking to students. Several participants stated that they sometimes did not recognize bullying at the time they experienced it. They stated that it was how the behaviors made them feel that resulted in them labeling it as bullying, rather than the behaviors themselves. Participants said bullying made them feel that their presence was not wanted or was unnecessary. One participant stated that bullying "makes you feel degraded as a human being" (p. 49).

Tanner-Garrett (2014) found the most apparent theme to be the devaluing of students by others. The message of "You're just a student" was described by several participants, who also shared comments that they had overheard from physicians or nursing staff, such as "Well, get the *student* [emphasis added] to do it! The *student* [emphasis added] can go clean up that patient" (p. 51). Students were often expected to complete tasks that others did not want to do, yet were sometimes denied the opportunity to participate in new procedures because they were students. A participant described one situation in which a physician ordered others to "Get all the students out of the room, they don't need to be in here, they're just students, there's no reason for them to be in here taking up space!" (p. 51). Tanner-Garrett (2014) categorized this devaluing as "less than." When the students internalized the "less than" belief, they described feeling trapped. One participant described this:

> As a student, you don't know the facility, you don't know
> who to go talk to, you don't know, hey, if I stand up for
> myself, or tell them "Hey, you can't talk to me this way...."
> Then, I mean, obviously, they work here and you don't,
> so obviously, you're below them in a sense, and...so it's
> like, uh-oh, you're stuck. Like a catch-22. It was horrible.
> (Tanner-Garrett, 2014, p. 56)

The devaluing of students was often communicated by ignoring them. One student described this, "You'd walk up to the desk and acknowledge the nurses like you always do and they wouldn't even look at you, wouldn't acknowledge you, wouldn't make an effort to try to engage with you or try to help you in any way" (p. 52). Another participant stated, "they would sigh if you asked them something, like... 'You're bothering me'" (p. 52). Students described their embarrassment at being ignored in front of patients, which also affected their learning.

It was clear from participants in the Tanner-Garrett (2014) study that bullying often leads to squandered learning experiences. The experience of being ignored, marginalized, or belittled affected their interactions with those who were bullying them and they often felt shut out of experiences that they believed would have helped them learn. One participant stated, "I wanted to see the chest tube placed...and the doctor wouldn't let me watch, because I was a student. He only wanted the nurse to be in there, because there 'wasn't any reason for me to see that'" (p. 52). Another participant recalled, "There was one rotation where I stood at the desk most of the time and I would have to, like, stay on this nurse's coattails to make sure I got to do anything" (p. 53). Participants described their frustration that they were wasting time instead of being able to participate in experiences that would have fostered learning and understanding of the role of a nurse.

Perhaps one of the most poignant findings in the Tanner-Garrett (2014) study was that the experience of bullying often caused students to question their choice of nursing as a career. One participant stated,

> It made me feel like this wasn't something I wanted to
> be a part of, if that's how I was going to be treated. Once
> I became a nurse, why would I put myself through this,
> because it's very stressful. It made me question whether
> nursing was the right choice for me...it definitely made
> me question myself at the time, like "Did I make the right
> decision? Is nursing the correct area for me? If this is how
> nurses act all the time, if this is how doctors treat nurses
> all the time, is this what I should really be doing? Is this
> really worth it, is it gonna be worth it in the future?"
> (Tanner-Garrett, 2014, p. 59)

Research suggests that faculty are not the primary source of student bullying—it comes more often from nurses or physicians on the hospital units. In the Tanner-Garrett (2014) study, only two participants reported bullying from faculty. One student commented, "Well, they tell us that nurses eat their young, and maybe this is what they're talking about" (p. 6). This has important implications for clinical nurse educators, in that they not only need to ensure that they interact with students in a caring way, but they also are watchful for any bullying behaviors on the part of nurses and other staff. Researchers in one study found that 36% of clinical educators surveyed reported difficulty when confronted with incivility, suggesting a need for additional information and guidance for working with students in this area (Suplee, Gardner, & Jerome-D'Emilia, 2014). Clinical nurse educators may want to have an open discussion with their students about this problem, such as devoting a clinical post conference to the issue. In this way, faculty and students can talk together about incivility experiences they have had and possible interventions to remediate the problem.

Research has shown that bullying of nursing students is underreported, often because students fear retaliation. In a study of 313 second- and third-year nursing students from a large school of nursing in the United Kingdom, 53% of the students stated that they had experienced bullying behaviors (Stevenson, Randle, & Grayling, 2006). Over 100 students in the sample took no action related to it, stating that they knew they had very little power so it was difficult to challenge negative behaviors directed toward them from persons of authority. Various studies have demonstrated that bullying has serious effects on students, including such problems as increased stress, reduced self-esteem and confidence, reduced ability to learn, increased absences, anxiety, and intention to leave the profession (Clark, 2008; Stevenson et al., 2006; Tanner-Garrett, 2014). Researchers have also found that students' perceptions of bullying change over time; initially students expressed shock at bullying behaviors but came to see that this behavior appeared to be accepted in the nursing profession—certainly not the message we want to give students.

REFLECTIONS FOR NEW NURSE EDUCATORS

Even though faculty seldom talk about their "power," it is clear from the stories in this chapter that faculty have a great deal of power to create experiences for students—hopefully positive experiences—that they will remember for a long time. The stories help to illustrate Van Manen's concept of the tact of teaching. According to Van Manen (1991), "Tact derives etymologically from the Latin tactus, meaning touch, effect... tactful means fully in touch, and it also suggests being able to have an effect" (p. 126). This concept can help new clinical nurse educators use their power to provide a caring learning environment for their students. Van Manen (1991) stated that it is important to offer a caring and supportive environment, not only because a caring teaching approach tends to reproduce a caring orientation in the students themselves, but also because this approach fosters a climate for personal growth (pp. 34–35).

Van Manen (1991) used the word "pedagogy" to refer, not to curricular aspects of structure, phases, and objectives, but to the human or personal elements of education. Pedagogy encompasses a wide range of teacher and student relations that create a personal learning relationship with active and meaningful encounters between teacher and student. Van Manen (1991) called these interactions "pedagogical moments"— a specific encounter when the teacher can make an important difference for student learning (p. 40). Carrie's experience—when the nurse took the time to find her after her patient died in order to assure her that she had not done anything wrong—illustrates the power of the pedagogical moment.

Using pedagogical moments effectively means that the teacher will have an intuitive sense of pedagogical tact that creates thoughtful actions toward others (Van Manen, 1991). Van Manen (1991) noted that to be tactful means to touch someone in a meaningful way, whether with a word, a gesture, action, or with silence (pp. 142–143). This approach to teaching can lead to an embodied knowing that is based not in textbook teaching strategies but in knowing how to create student–teacher interactions for learning. The student does not merely learn facts but *experiences* knowing. Pedagogical tact cannot be false or feigned, and any influence the teacher has on the student that is mediated by tact "is not authoritarian, controlling, dominating or manipulative" (Van Manen, 1991, p. 161). This approach to teaching usually requires a type of tactful action that is essentially unplanned because it is an integral part of a caring approach to teaching, the expression of a thoughtful and mindful approach toward meeting the needs of the other person (Van Manen, 1991, p. 146).

Faculty need to consciously assess what words and actions are appropriate with their students and then communicate them to the students in a caring manner. The concept of tact in teaching will motivate teachers to ask themselves how they can interact best with their students to help them understand. According to Van Manen (1991), meaningful teaching consists of pedagogical moments that reflect thoughtfulness and tact. To teach with tact, the teacher needs to *see* a situation calling for sensitivity, *understand* the meaning of the situation, *sense* the significance of the situation and what to do, and *act* in a way that is right (p. 146). Through the blending of expertise and thoughtful practice, a teacher can transform an unproductive situation into a critical learning experience for the student.

Creating a Caring Learning Environment

A clinical nurse educator who is new to the role can use this information to create a caring learning environment that will help students to feel empowered and will support their learning. Three concepts help to illustrate how clinical nurse educators can do this: (a) *caring as offering*; (b) *leaps ahead caring*; and (c) *creating a caring place* (Sorrell & Redmond, 1997).

Caring as Offering. Studies of students' perceptions of caring have demonstrated that students view faculty members and other staff as authority figures. Students may feel intimidated by the knowledge level of faculty and feel that faculty are "too smart to bring it down to the students' level" (Clark, 2006). Clinical instructors can be very helpful by offering themselves to the students as not only persons who impart knowledge and evaluate, but also as sounding boards for issues of concern and a resource to help students move through difficult situations. The caring stories of Nancy and Carrie illustrate how important it is for students to have someone offer him- or herself to students. It is important for students to see the clinical instructor as a learner, too. Sharing instructors' own concerns with students will help students see that instructors are vulnerable, too. It is important for nurse educators to model caring relationships in order to create a caring learning environment for students (Labrague, McEnroe-Petitte, Papathanasiou, Edet, & Arulappan, 2015).

Leaps Ahead Caring. Heidegger (1962, pp. 158–159) used the term "leap" to convey a type of forethinking or intuitive knowing that can cause one to leap beyond familiar patterns of behavior to enter into the realm of another being. The concept of "leaps ahead caring" is reflected in students' stories of caring where sometimes faculty knew what students needed before students themselves knew. An example is one student who shared her experience of caring for an elderly aphasic patient who seemed to be ignored by staff because she could not communicate verbally. The student was angry at the staff but tried not to show it because she wanted to act professionally. Nevertheless, her instructor sensed her real feelings and encouraged her to talk about them. The student said,

> He noticed something different about me, because I'm
> usually a very "up" person. I felt so guilty for not say-
> ing anything. He purposefully assigned me to her again.
> I know he did, and I was able to work through that... to
> make peace with myself about the guilt. He told me, "You
> know, that's something that comes with time, you'll learn

to assert yourself. You need to forgive yourself." (Sorrell & Redmond, 1997, p. 231)

New clinical educators may not have the experience to sense when a student needs help, but just as for students, this will come with time. The important thing is to be aware of the possibility for the need to step in to help a student interpret a difficult situation, even before the student may sense the need for help.

Creating a Caring Place. The clinical context can be a stressful environment for any health care professional, but especially for students and new nurses. They are thrust into an environment of pain, intimacy, uncertainty, and confusion that may seem overwhelming to them. Many times students may have unclear expectations of the nursing education experience (Hoffman, 2012). This is one area where you can be uniquely helpful. You already have the clinical experience that makes you feel comfortable with patients, other nurses, physicians, and other clinical staff. Thus, you can use your confidence to help the students and new nurses face their anxiety and fears, creating a safe haven for both personal and professional learning. Students and novice nurses may not be able to see the whole picture of a situation, and instead may focus on parts of the picture that are right in front of them. They are often fearful of making mistakes that may harm patients and feel unsure about how to transfer their learning from the classroom to nursing care for their patients. You can help them make this transition by creating a caring environment where they feel free to ask questions, know that you are there to support them, and feel confident that you will step in as needed if they make a mistake. In this way, you function both as a coach and as someone who helps empower the student or new nurse to act in the patient's best interest.

Strategies for Creating a Caring Environment for Learning

- Listen actively to students to learn their expectations and concerns.
- Convey to students a genuine interest and concern for them as individuals and for their learning needs.
- Provide clear explanations of what you expect from students and encourage their feedback related to these explanations.

- Schedule individual conferences for students to share perspectives on their experiences and discuss problems they have encountered; schedule group conferences to help students learn to give and receive support from peers and faculty.
- Structure opportunities for discussion of experiences related to incivility that the students may have encountered.
- Implement creative clinical assignments, such as weekly journals, to encourage student reflection and sharing of concerns.
- Consider cultural influences with your students that may affect their learning.
- Establish effective working relationships with staff members who interact with your students and encourage them to discuss issues of concern with you.

The National League for Nursing (NLN) Competency No. 2 notes the importance of creating learning environments that are focused on socialization to the role of the nurse and facilitate students' self-reflection and personal goal setting (NLN, 2005). NLN Competency No. 5 calls for the nurse educator to model cultural sensitivity when advocating for change. Many current changes in the educational process for nursing students, such as increased class size, clinical experiences spread across different institutions within the community, and a shortage of clinical faculty, make it more difficult for the new clinical nurse educator to know how to meet these competencies. Stories of students and faculty experiences can help clinical educators recognize the responsibility and power that they have to establish thoughtful and tactful connections with their students to create a caring learning environment.

Questions for Reflection

1. One of your students tells you that he overheard one of the staff nurses saying to another nurse that she wished they did not have students on the unit every week. What would you do?
2. You notice that Sumiko, an ESL student from Japan, never makes any comments during your post conference on the unit. She often "hangs out" in the library on the unit when she is not with her assigned patient. What do you think might be the

reason for her behavior? What could you do to create a caring environment?

3. At a faculty meeting, one of the faculty members complains that faculty have no power and that she is sick and tired of her concerns not being heard. How could you engage her in conversation about this?

4. One student writes in her journal that she feels frightened and incompetent during her clinical time on the cardiac unit. How would you respond?

REFERENCES

Allen, J., Brown, L., Duff, C., Nesbitt, P., & Hepner, A. (2013). Development and evaluation of a teaching and learning approach in cross-cultural care and antidiscrimination in university nursing students. *Nurse Education Today, 33*(12), 1592–1598.

Clark, C. M. (2006). *Incivility in nursing education: Student perceptions of uncivil faculty behavior in the academic environment.* (Doctoral dissertation). Retrieved from ProQuest Dissertations & Theses Global. (3216197.)

Clark, C. M. (2008). The dance of incivility in nursing education as described by nursing faculty and students. *Advances in Nursing Science, 31*(4), 37–54.

Crawford, T., & Candlin, S. (2013). Investigating the language needs of culturally and linguistically diverse nursing students to assist their completion of the bachelor of nursing programme to become safe and effective practitioners. *Nurse Education Today, 33,* 796–801.

Davis, S. P., Davis, D. D., & Williams, D. D. (2010). Challenges and issues facing the future of nursing education: Implications for ethnic minority faculty and students. *Journal of Cultural Diversity, 17*(4), 122–126.

Fitzsimmons, K. A. (2009). *The existence of implicit racial bias in nursing faculty.* (Doctoral dissertation). Retrieved from ProQuest Dissertations & Theses Global. (3397096.)

Glasgow, F. (2014). *Cultural sensitivity: Voices of nursing faculty and entry-level ESL students.* (Doctoral study). Retrieved from ProQuest Dissertations & Theses Global. (3621830.)

Harvey, T., Robinson, C., & Frohman, R. (2013). Preparing culturally and linguistically diverse nursing students for clinical practice in the health care setting. *Journal of Nursing Education, 52*(7), 365–370.

Heidegger, M. (1962). *Being and time* (J. Macquarrie & E. Robinson, Trans.). New York: Harper & Row. (Original work published 1927).

Hoffman, R. L. (2012). *Differences in student perceptions of student and faculty incivility among nursing program types: An application of attribution theory.* (Doctoral dissertation). Retrieved from ProQuest Dissertations & Theses Global. (3547431.)

Labrague, L. J., McEnroe-Petitte, D. M., Papathanasiou, I. V., Edet, O. B., & Arulappan, J. (2015). Impact of instructors' caring on students' perceptions of their own caring behaviors. *Journal of Nursing Scholarship, 47*, 338–346.

Long, T. B. (2012). Overview of teaching strategies for cultural competence in nursing students. *Journal of Cultural Diversity, 19*(3), 102–108.

National League for Nursing. (2005). *Core competencies of nurse educators with task statements.* Retrieved from www.nln.org/profdev/corecompetencies.pdf

Redmond, G. M., & Sorrell, J. M. (1996). Creating a caring learning environment. *Nursing Forum, 31*(4), 21–27.

Sorrell, J. M., & Redmond, G. M. (1997). The lived experiences of students in nursing: Voices of caring speak of the tact of teaching. *Journal of Professional Nursing, 13*(4), 228–235.

Stevenson, K., Randle, J., & Grayling, I. (2006). Inter-group health care conflict: UK students' experiences of bullying and the need for organizational solutions. *Online Journal of Issues in Nursing, 11*(2), 3–12. Retrieved from www.nursingworld.org/OJIN

Suplee, P. D., Gardner, M., & Jerome-D'Emilia, B. (2014) Nursing faculty preparedness for clinical teaching. *Journal of Nursing Education, 53*(3, Suppl.), S38–S41.

Tanner-Garrett, M. (2014). *Recent female graduate nurses' experiences with bullying.* (Doctoral study). Retrieved from ProQuest Dissertations & Theses Global. (3630525.)

Van Manen, M. (1991). *The tact of teaching: The meaning of pedagogical thoughtfulness.* Albany, NY: State University of New York Press.

CHAPTER 4

Clinical Evaluation of Students: Where Does Learning Stop and Evaluation Begin?

One instructor ... would yell and belittle us in front of the other students. ... I firmly believe that all people need to feel respected and valued.

—Hannah

I was in my first weeks of clinical as a nursing student. I was young and inexperienced in talking to patients, and very shy. I was assigned to give a bed bath to an elderly man and was very nervous about remembering all the steps I had learned in the skills lab. I concentrated intently on folding the washcloth the right way, making sure that the water in the washbasin was the right temperature, and keeping the patient covered with a bath blanket while doing the bath so that he would not feel cold. I thought the procedure went well and the patient thanked me warmly for my care.

Later that day, my instructor called me into the confer-ence room to talk. "I was watching outside the curtain this morning when you were bathing your patient," she said. "Maybe you don't realize it, but you hardly said a word to him the whole time. You are supposed to be using therapeutic communication during the procedure, not just going through the motions of the bath. You seem to have difficulty communicating. Maybe you should think about a career other than nursing."

This incident happened many years ago. The student to whom it happened was me, one of the co-authors. I was shocked that I had been judged so soon and so harshly. The incident made me so angry that I determined I would *not* give this instructor the satisfaction of my leaving nursing. But the story could have ended differently. After many years of clinical nursing and teaching, I have never forgotten the experience and how I felt. I wonder how many other students or new graduates, struggling to gain confidence and competence in the clinical area, withdraw from nursing because of too harsh judgment that comes too soon.

THE STORIES

Many nurse educators consider clinical teaching the most difficult part of the nurse educator role. And the most difficult part of clinical teaching may be the process of clinical evaluation of students. It is the clinical instructor's responsibility not only to keep the students' patients safe, providing them with excellent nursing care, but also to facilitate the students' learning. Thus, the instructor constantly moves between responsibilities to the patients and the students—and also the nursing and medical staff on the unit, who have the ultimate responsibility for the patients' care. It is critical to create a learning environment where students feel comfortable and also to monitor students' progress to ensure that they are practicing responsibly.

Students need time to learn new skills and they learn at different rates and in different ways. If students are slow learners, should they be given more time to demonstrate satisfactory performance than students who appear to learn required skills readily? Perhaps given adequate time for learning, these students will eventually be successful. Or should the instructor be able to know early on whether a student will succeed? If an instructor allows "weak" students to progress into the next course, hoping that they will eventually gain the needed skills, how long should these students be allowed to continue? Is it fair to allow students to progress almost to graduation and then decide that they cannot pass and must leave the program? Or is it better to decide early that a particular student will not succeed?

These are all difficult questions for even an experienced nurse educator to answer. And for novice educators, clinical evaluation of students can be a scary and challenging process. Stories in the following sections from participants in the Clinical Nurse Educator Academy illustrate the difficulty of the evaluation process for novice nurse educators, as well as my own, along with the importance of the process for students' learning (Cangelosi, Crocker, & Sorrell, 2009). The stories are focused around important aspects of carrying out clinical evaluations: respect, communication, a safe learning environment, collaborative goal development, and helping students see the big picture of their role as students moving toward professional nursing practice.

Respect for Persons and Different Processes of Learning

It is important to remember that you may feel like a novice as an educator, but for the student, the feeling of being a novice in the clinical environment may be overwhelming. Fear may keep students from performing as they would once they have more confidence. It is important to assure students that you respect their individual differences in learning and that you will guide them toward situations that will help them build self-confidence. Hannah, a nurse participating in the nurse academy whose comment is at the beginning of this chapter, noted a critical element that should be part of any clinical evaluation—respect for the student as a person and as a learner:

> Changing roles from an expert clinician to a novice nurse
> educator definitely will cause me to self-reflect.... I think
> about all of the instructors I had during my clinical experi-
> ences and none were perfect. I am not sure there is such
> a thing, yet I have learned from all of them. Each instruc-
> tor had valuable information to share. I was eager for the
> knowledge. I watched and absorbed every little detail.
>   There was only one instructor who left a negative
> impression in my memory. I will never forget her as she

was extremely critical of all of the students and made us feel inferior. She would yell and belittle us in front of the other students.... I firmly believe that all people need to feel respected and valued.

Since most beginning students and new graduate nurses feel very vulnerable in the unfamiliar clinical environment, what they perceive as a lack of respect from an instructor can have a profound impact on their self-confidence. Cara's memories of an incident where she felt a lack of respect from faculty have stayed with her for many years:

During my senior year, I overheard a group of three nursing faculty discussing and laughing about a particular student's actions.... My respect for those instructors diminished. I felt badly for the student whose name they mentioned. We were all working so hard and looking for guidance. That could have been any one of us. We were students who were searching for role models to help mentor us and teach us about what it means to be a nurse. I was shocked by such unprofessional behavior exhibited by the esteemed faculty I had highly respected. I knew I didn't want to be that type of nurse.

Respect for individuals and their learning styles includes the need to apply standards in a way that allows for individual variation. Sabrina noted the importance of a nonjudgmental attitude:

I think being nonjudgmental is a critical trait.... You need to encourage students to ask questions and be honest about their capabilities and areas for growth. If you are judgmental, you will shut students down and they may get into trouble.

As a clinical educator, you work closely with individual students and new graduate nurses, so you are in an excellent position to see qualities and limitations in them that others might not see. You want them to feel at their best when their performance is being evaluated. You can make an important difference by pointing out to an individual a particular strength that you note. For example, Lisa commented: *I had an RN supervisor who saw in me something I was not aware I possess—leadership abilities.* When you see yourself not merely as someone to judge the students or new graduates, but as someone who is there to help them recognize their strengths and limitations, you will also feel more comfortable in your novice educator role, as students will see you as someone to guide them, not to judge them.

Compassionate and Constructive Communication

In the fast-paced clinical environment, it is easy to lose sight of how important it is to take time to communicate with students and new graduate nurses about how you view their performance on a continuum of learning. The educator must be observant and intuitive to know the best time to communicate this information. It is also important to deliver the message compassionately, respecting the student's right to privacy and dignity. Cara described an incident when she did not receive the explanations she needed about her performance of giving an injection. It is evident that the incident impacted her ability to feel confident about her learning:

> I remember back to my days in clinical education when everything revolved around the nursing faculty. They sat upon that pedestal where everything they did you believed was worth role modeling. The atmosphere was not one that facilitated or fostered new or creative ideas. You did it their way or you failed. I remember my first IM [intramuscular] injection; the instructor grabbed my hand and assisted me. I felt disheartened. There was no communication from the instructor if I was doing something wrong or if she did that with all nurses on their first shot. How frustrated I was, never knowing what she was going to do to me next.

Perhaps the instructor meant to be helpful by reaching in to assist with the injection. But it is clear from Cara's description of the incident that she needed more feedback from the instructor about how she was doing and what she should do differently next time. Students who do not receive helpful feedback from teachers may compare themselves too harshly with those who are more advanced in their studies. This may lead to a level of decreased self-confidence that may have a negative impact on clinical performance (Plakht, Shiyovich, Nusbaum, & Raizer, 2013).

Creating a Safe Environment for Mistakes

It is important for students and new graduate nurses to realize that everyone makes mistakes but that it is important to address the errors and learn from them. I once observed a clinical instructor warning her students about the dangers of making a medication error. She warned the students: "If I ever made a medication error, I think I would have to leave nursing." Her comments sent chills through me, as I had already made several medication errors in my practice. Fortunately, they had not created serious harm and I learned a great deal from my errors. But how would these students feel if they made a medication error? Would the instructor's words stay with them to create a serious lack of self-confidence or even cause them to leave nursing?

In the process of clinical evaluation, it is important not only to point out errors that a student or nurse may be making but also to help them see how to remedy the situation. If individuals fear that by reporting an error they will be punished, they may hide their error. Thus, it is important to create a learning environment that feels safe for communicating errors when they occur. Cara emphasized this, calling out for a "safe harbor" for learning:

> I think for any learning to take place you have to create a safe environment. This includes respecting students as people.... Once a safe harbor is provided, students feel more at ease that their character will not be judged or torn down. Providing a safe environment allows the student to feel more at ease in coming to you and asking questions. If I know a student is performing a skill for the first time, together we review the steps in that procedure. Depending on the comfort level of the student, he or she may only need me there for support and to catch them if they should stumble. Other students need to focus and think totally about the skill while I will talk with the patient. This is being in tune with their verbal and nonverbal communication.

In the process of creating a safe environment for students, it is important to consider how assessment from clinical nurses on the unit may affect students. Clinicians who have many years of vast experience may forget how much they had to learn along the way and may be impatient with students who do not seem to be mastering skills quickly enough. As the nurse educator on the unit, it is helpful to develop a positive relationship with the staff, including them in your goals for the students. Lynn pointed out how she addresses this:

> I may have to stand up for my students if issues arise with staff or patients. I want to listen, understand, encourage, and support my students. To put it best, I want to be available.

One educator described a very disturbing incident that had happened with a student on a neurosurgical unit where the head nurse did not want students, but was required to have them by the hospital supervisor:

> I was responsible for two different groups of students on two different floors so I had to run up and down the stairs often to make sure that I was available when students needed me. At one point, I walked on to the neuro unit to see a patient's gown being hurled into the hallway as the head nurse stormed out and marched down the hall to the nurses' station. My student, standing by the patient's bed, looked as if he were in shock. When I took him aside to find out what had happened, he explained that the patient, who was being evaluated for a possible sub-arachnoid hemorrhage, was on complete bed rest. He had completed the bed bath and then helped his patient into a clean gown. When the head nurse entered, she was furious, saying that the student did not understand what complete bed rest meant and that he had possibly caused harm by allowing the patient to move around in bed.
>
> This explanation seemed to make no sense at all. Surely there must have been some other rationale for why the head nurse had acted toward the student as she had. I tried to get an explanation from her but she just walked away. I felt that I needed to protect future students from such harsh behavior so I reported the incident to the hospital supervisor, who seemed appreciative that I had brought it to her attention. The supervisor scheduled a conference for her, the head nurse, and me to discuss the situation. On the day scheduled for the conference, I was terrified

at the prospect of confronting this nurse again! But at the last minute, she called the supervisor to say something had come up on the unit and she wouldn't be able to get away to meet with me. I never saw her again.

Developing Collaborative Goals

It is important for students to know your expectations of what they should accomplish in a course, but it also is important for you to know students' individual goals that they want to meet. As a clinical nurse educator, you will be responsible for guiding students to meet objectives for the course. However, course objectives are broad and meant to apply to all students in the course. It is important to remember that students are each at a different learning point in the course and set different goals for themselves. I remember one clinical group of new students that I took to a nursing home for their first experience. I had them wait in the hallway while I went in the room of an elderly man to see if he would agree to have me bring in the students to talk with him. After chatting with him a few minutes, I returned to the student group to tell them it would be fine for us to go into the patient's room. One student stared at me, amazed. "How do you do that?" she asked. "How do I do what?" I responded, confused by her question. "Talk to a stranger like that! How do you know what to say when you go into a stranger's room like that? I don't think I can ever do that!"

This incident helped me remember that many young students have never been in situations where they have to interact in a health professional–patient role and that many are even unfamiliar with relating to older adults. This student's response made me realize that one goal I needed to help her with that semester was to feel comfortable in initiating focused communications with different patients—and she did accomplish this!

Students are used to articulating their goals in formal terms, as required in many of their classes. But as in the incident just described, students often have personal goals that they want to meet, for example, to enhance their confidence and skill in therapeutic communication, gain an understanding of cultural aspects of patient care, or improve organizational skills in caring for more than one patient at a time. It is important to structure opportunities for sharing these individual goals. Cara described how she approached this with her students:

> Providing clear guidelines, direction, and support are other teaching methods students need. Students, like adult learners, use stories and lessons learned to aid in their own growth. It is amazing to see the light bulbs go on; those "a-ha" moments. During one of my evaluation summaries from nursing students this past year, they requested more real-life stories from clinical practice. They enjoy sharing their clinical stories in post conference. Students learn as they teach one another. They are able to benefit from the clinical experiences of others.
>
> A goal of mine is to determine how much room the student needs to grow without feeling smothered. The difficult part, the real art of teaching, is finding that magic balance between giving them enough information to make their own discoveries without handing them everything on a silver platter. Providing students with small steps of freedom in their new practice provides them with an increasing self-confidence and reassurance that they are acquiring necessary and useful skills.

Cara was very wise in knowing that the art of teaching requires "finding the magic balance between giving them enough information to make their own discoveries without handing them everything on a silver platter" and "providing students with small steps of freedom" for success.

Jolene described how one clinical educator in the hospital made it possible for a new nurse to succeed by sharing goals and developing individual learning plans:

> A few years ago, new hire nurses were assigned to a clinical nurse mentor for orientation. This orientation was structured to be accomplished within 1 year, with the goal of producing a fully functioning clinical nurse. One of the new hires was an older nurse returning to patient care after several years of working in risk management. She was enthusiastic, pleasant, and a team player. The challenges arose when the orientation program schedule exceeded her individual learning pace. The imposed requirements of

attending the didactic lecture sessions, applying the nursing clinical skills, and managing patient charts became a source of difficulty and frustration for her. In addition, administering immunizations to infants and small children, in particular, seemed to be an obstacle that caused her anxiety.

Her clinical nurse mentor took steps to help her. Through individualized meetings, each concern and problem was identified. Then, they jointly worked on each issue. This new hire successfully completed the orientation program because her mentor took additional time for one-on-one clinical instruction. She provided her with extra appropriate materials and videos, and gave her encouragement. Recognizing that each individual is unique and that learning occurs differently were two key factors to restructuring and extending her orientation. She became a valuable clinic team member and enjoyed her new experiences in patient care.

Framing the Learning

One very helpful teaching strategy to think about in clinical evaluation is to help students see the "big picture" of their learning over time. They may be too critical of themselves, upset that they do not know what they need to know. It is important to reassure them that learning is not a linear, time-limited process—they will build upon their learning, course by course, and even after graduation.

Nurse educators who are orienting new graduate nurses in a hospital or other setting face problems similar to nurse educators in a school of nursing. They are responsible for assessing competency of the nurses, and also need to reassure the nurses that they will be allowed adequate time to master new skills. Lynn shared the following memory of her experience as a new graduate and how important it is to know there will be more opportunities for learning, hopefully positive ones, after graduation:

> I remember thinking: My nursing program is supposed to be one of the best schools in the state, so I should have learned all I needed to know ... right? I even passed my NCLEX exam the first time; I'm adequately prepared as a nurse ... don't you think? But as I started my new career as

a nursery/NICU/delivery room nurse, I realized that there was a lot I did not know. I had only one pediatric rotation, although I did have the opportunity to do my practicum in a pediatric clinic. I felt comfortable with one thing: giving shots. The rest of it was news to me.

I must admit, that this was very disturbing for me. I'm the kind of person that likes to know everything upfront before I do it.... I felt like a nursing student all over again. Thank goodness the nurses on my unit didn't "eat their young." I was fortunate enough to have two good preceptors during my orientation. They were patient, kind, understanding, yet firm. That was exactly what I needed. I definitely wouldn't say I was an expert by the end of orientation, but these nurses did lay a good foundation for me to one day acquire that status—which of course, after only 5 years as a nurse, I have yet to reach!

Cara offered the following reflection on her feelings about the responsibility of helping new graduates transition successfully into their new clinical roles:

I accepted a nursing position in an acute care facility....
I began my job there shortly before eight new graduate nurses started and quickly realized I was mentoring these new nurses in their transition from student to nurse. I had concerns about these nurses entering a specialty area without having first learned basic nursing practice. These nurses were given approximately 6 months of orientation. Orientation consisted of a little classroom theory along with being placed with a mentor who may have been there 1 or more years. Many concerns raced through my head, including the safety of the patients and the staff, and legal issues, including medication administration.

My concerns were: How are we going to give these nurses the time and experiences they need to grow in a fast-paced unit where everything seems like an emergency? How am I going to bridge these new graduates from novices to functioning competent nurses?... I felt responsible for these nurses. I wanted them to have a positive experience and stay engaged in nursing. There are so many things to consider in training new graduate nurses, such as providing them with evidence-based practice and fostering time management skills as well as being a professional role model for them. Promoting trust in new graduate nurses is also difficult. Sometimes it's difficult to know when to step in so they learn skills and not flounder, always thinking about safety for both the patient and the nurse.

Cara's concluding thought—"Sometimes it's difficult to know when to step in so they learn skills and not flounder, always thinking about safety for both the patient and the nurse"—captures the essence of the tightrope on which the nurse educator balances when teaching students or new graduates.

REFLECTIONS FOR NEW NURSE EDUCATORS

Clinical evaluation is a complex skill that involves evaluation of such factors as students' knowledge, understanding, problem solving, critical thinking, technical skills, attitudes, ethics, appropriate professional behavior, appropriate interaction with the patients, and ability to prioritize problems (Rafiee, Moattari, Nikbakht, Kojuri, & Mousavinasab, 2014; Zafrir & Nissim, 2011). The evaluation process involves collecting and analyzing multiple observations regarding students' abilities and transforming these data into an evaluation that is objective and meaningful to students (Zafrir & Nissim, 2011).

It is surprising that, since clinical evaluation is such an important part of clinical teaching, there is not more research related to what approaches to evaluation are most effective for fostering learning. There are many different types of clinical evaluation tools described in the literature, along with a description of positive and negative aspects of the tools. Many nursing programs use tools developed specifically for their programs. As a new nurse educator, you will probably be required to use a tool for evaluating your students that is provided to you. Perhaps more important than the tool, however, is the process by which you use the tool to evaluate the competency of your students. A consideration of the culture of the clinical unit, research related to students' perceptions of the evaluation process, the need for formative evaluation with constructive feedback, and factors to consider in passing or failing a student can help you feel more confident about your evaluation of students and also enhance their learning.

Culture of the Clinical Unit

Activities on the clinical unit of a hospital are primarily focused on provision of care for patients, that is, performing tasks, with teaching and learning being a "secondary" activity (Henderson & Eaton, 2013). Thus, when you bring students into a clinical unit for learning, it is important to think about how you will integrate teaching and learning for your students into this culture. In some sense, you are a "guest" in the unit organization and need to have an understanding of its culture.

If you are not familiar with the unit, it is often helpful for you to spend some time there before students begin their clinical rotation so that you know the layout of the unit and the personnel. Research has shown that effective clinical evaluation integrates data from multiple situations and observers, so you want to be able to integrate data obtained from staff on the unit, as well as your own observations. Establish a relationship with nurses who provide the leadership for the unit and share with them your goals for students' learning. Assure nursing staff that you are aware of their primary role as caregivers and discuss with them their preferences for how you integrate your students into the workflow.

Nursing staff need to know details about placements of learners, such as the hours of attendance and the scope and entry-level skill of the student (Henderson & Eaton, 2013). What skills will the students be expected to demonstrate on the unit? Will they have "total care" of assigned patients or only partial care? Will they be giving medications? Who do they want the student to report to upon arriving and leaving the unit? These are the types of questions that will help you develop effective collaboration with unit staff and enhance continuity of care for the patients. If nursing staff have a poor understanding of the requirements of students, this can have a negative impact on learning experiences (Henderson & Eaton, 2013). When nurses know that you respect their primary responsibility for patient care and also know your goals for the students, a collaborative learning environment is fostered that encourages staff to work effectively with students and provide helpful feedback that is important for their evaluation.

Students' Perceptions of the Evaluation Process

Knowing how students and new graduate nurses perceive the assessment process can be helpful to you in implementing your clinical evaluations. However, there is little research focused on students' perceptions of the clinical evaluation process (McCutchan, 2010). There is even less research related to how new nurse graduates perceive evaluation of their competencies. The following studies, however, provide some beginning insights into how students perceive the evaluation process.

McCutchan (2010) focused her qualitative dissertation study on the experiences of baccalaureate nursing students undergoing clinical performance appraisals. Responses from interviews with nine senior students from two Midwest universities, six females and three males, revealed that students believed that the evaluation process was not consistent between instructors. Participants felt that there was disparity in instructor expectations, as well as individual interpretation of how the evaluation tool should be used to make a final grade determination. The majority of students felt that nurses on the unit who they had worked with should have input into the evaluation, since the instructor was often not there to see what they had done. Students saw the appraisal process as a formality, with no real connection to meeting their personal and professional goals. The most meaningful aspect of the evaluation process, however, was the dialogue with the instructor. One student described it this way:

> The part of the evaluation process that really does something for me is when I actually sit down with my professor because it's like, yeah, sure, I "meet" this meaningless sentence, but what does she see in me that she thinks would make me a good nurse? What does she see in me that I need to improve to be a better nurse? I mean, what do seasoned people see? You know, what would make me a bad nurse? And I think that helps me more than filling out, um, the meaningless sheet of paper. (McCutchan, 2010, p. 90)

Other studies that focused on student perceptions of the clinical evaluation process have uncovered similar concerns. A qualitative research study by Cazzell and Rodriguez (2011) focused on identifying feelings, beliefs, and attitudes of senior-level undergraduate pediatric nursing students after completion of an evaluation that included simulated medication administration in a skills lab. The authors noted that even though the affective domain is deemed the "gateway to learning," it is often neglected in higher education (Cazzell & Rodriguez, 2011, p. 711). The study included 20 students who responded to three questions:

- How would you describe the evaluation experience you completed? (feelings)
- What did you learn about yourself during this evaluation experience? (beliefs)
- What does this evaluation experience mean for you as you begin your capstone experience and your nursing career? (attitudes)

Regarding the first question, students expressed feelings of loss of control and anxiety due to unclear instructions and inconsistent involvement of staff during the simulation. Findings related to the second question identified two common beliefs of the students: their need for immediate feedback from the instructors as to how well they were performing and their need for instructors to understand that their reaction under pressure negatively affected their performance, preventing accurate assessment of their clinical competence in medication administration. Regarding the third question, many students' responses reflected the attitude that they could not make significant connections between the evaluation and their upcoming capstone experience or future nursing practice. They felt that the lack of immediate feedback from instructors was the primary reason for this inability to see connections in their learning.

Even though these were small studies, they point out important considerations for nurse educators in carrying out clinical evaluations. First, it is very important that students know "the rules" that will be used for the evaluation process: Who will be doing the evaluation? What factors will be evaluated? Will there be an opportunity for a "retake" if the first evaluation is poor? What impact will the evaluation have on the student's grade or performance review? It is also important that the process be implemented consistently for each of the instructor's students and between instructors. These considerations will help to decrease anxiety during the evaluation that may impede performance and result in an inaccurate assessment of actual competencies.

Another important consideration identified by the studies is the critical importance of immediate feedback. Students want and need frequent feedback to help them assess their own learning. Even if the course syllabus does not specify that formal formative evaluations will be a part of the assessment process, educators should provide feedback at various points during the course term to help students understand how they are progressing and what skills they need to focus on to achieve satisfactory competence by the end of the course.

Formative Evaluation With Constructive Feedback

The literature suggests that a good first clinical experience for students is a critical factor in helping to ensure a successful first year and beyond (Andrew, 2013). Students need both formative and summative clinical evaluation. Formative evaluation should be provided throughout the course, helping students to see the progress (or lack of it) that they are demonstrating. This enables them to compare the instructor's evaluation with their self-evaluation and discuss any discrepancies in the evaluation. Yet, most formal clinical evaluations are summative evaluations, done at the end of the course when students receive a grade for their performance (Plakht et al., 2013; Rafiee et al., 2014). At this point, the student no longer has an opportunity to improve performance. Thus, in your role as clinical evaluator, it is important to focus on not just the judgment of whether a student is passing or failing but to implement the evaluation process in such a way that students perceive it as a guide to help them progress successfully.

It is critically important for clinical educators to provide consistent and high-quality feedback to their students (Duffy, 2013). Plakht et al. (2013) implemented a study to assess the characteristics of feedback that nursing students received from their instructors during clinical experiences. The researchers identified the association of high- or low-quality feedback (as judged by the students) with students' clinical performance, self-evaluation, and contribution to their professional skills. Participants ($n = 124$) were third-year Israeli nursing students enrolled in an emergency nursing course between 2008 and 2010. Researchers found that high-quality *negative* feedback was associated with students' more accurate self-evaluation of their performance. High-quality *positive* feedback was associated with students' higher clinical performance, that is, students who felt that they were given better positive feedback delivered better care and received better grades for the course. However, the high-quality, positive feedback also appeared to cause students to overestimate their performance. It appears that effective self-evaluation starts with self-awareness and is strengthened when others, such as clinical instructors, peers, and patients, provide meaningful assessments (Plakht et al., 2013). Thus, by offering constructive feedback, both positive and negative, in formative evaluations, nurse educators can help students evaluate their own performance realistically.

Clinical evaluation requires continuous assessment throughout students' clinical rotation, where regular "snapshots" are taken of students' practice and feedback is given frequently both formally and informally (Duffy, 2013). Although it is clear that students need regular feedback on their clinical performance, many nurse educators do not feel confident in doing this (Duffy, 2013). One of the most difficult tasks for clinical educators is to provide constructive feedback, especially when it is negative feedback (Plakht et al., 2013).

Boxes 4.1 and 4.2 provide examples of positive and negative constructive feedback.

BOX 4.1: EXAMPLE OF POSITIVE CONSTRUCTIVE FEEDBACK

I was happy to see how well you engaged Mr. Jones in talking about his experiences with diabetes today. The information you provided him about timing his insulin with his meals was excellent. You also took time to sit down with him, maintain eye contact, and make sure that he felt free to ask questions. This approach fit so well with our unit this week on patient teaching. Nice job!

BOX 4.2: EXAMPLE OF NEGATIVE CONSTRUCTIVE FEEDBACK

I noticed that you spent quite a lot of time today teaching Mr. Jones about his diabetes. This fits well with our focus on patient teaching this week. I have some suggestions though that would make your teaching more effective. Take time to sit down next to him when you are talking, so that he feels comfortable in asking questions. It is good to find out first from him what concerns he has, rather than just give him textbook-type information. You have limited time for teaching so you want to address the areas that are most important to him. Also, it would be good to use "teach-back" techniques, having him tell you what he understands about the information you have given him. I think you have a good start on teaching your patients about their care!

When providing feedback, it is helpful to use "I" statements, especially when providing negative feedback. Using "you" in such situations can make the student feel blame. As the instructor, you want to take responsibility, express your feelings, and let the student know how his or her behavior has affected you (Duffy, 2013). It is also helpful to use a "sandwich" approach by inserting the negative feedback in the middle of your comments. Students may not "hear" your message if you only provide negative feedback or make them feel blame. Starting and ending your comments with an observation of a positive behavior will help them from feeling completely incompetent and help to encourage more positive behaviors in the future.

Passing or Failing

One of the most difficult decisions for a nurse educator is whether to pass or fail a student in the clinical area. One reason that decisions can be difficult is that clinical evaluation tools are often mechanistic and derived from broad course learning outcomes; they frequently do not reflect specific clinical behaviors that determine success or failure or address the various interpretations of human behavior in the clinical environment (DeBrew & Lewallen, 2014; Diekelmann & McGregor, 2003). Research has shown that educators have difficulty in recognizing in a timely manner those students who need to fail (Heaslip & Scammell, 2012).

DeBrew and Lewallen (2014) implemented a qualitative study to explore factors that educators consider in making a decision to pass or fail a student in a clinical course. They asked 24 nurse educators from a variety of nursing programs in one southeastern state to describe critical incidents that they experienced in deciding whether to pass or fail a student. The most common reason for failing students was that faculty judged the student as a poor communicator, either verbally or in writing, and with patients, faculty, and staff nurses. The second most common reason for failing a student was the judgment that the student was not progressing in meeting course objectives, even after faculty tried to help by creating a learning contract or devoting extra time with the student. Other important factors for failing students were unsafe medication administration, inability to prioritize patient care, lack of preparedness, unprofessional behavior, personal problems, and academic integrity issues.

DeBrew and Lewallen (2014) noted that using the term "process" for clinical evaluation may be a misnomer. Findings from their study showed that faculty did not use a standardized procedure for decisions to pass or fail. Instead, they reacted to specific student characteristics and behaviors and drew from their past experiences in making their decisions. Findings from this study supported findings from previous studies that suggest that decisions to pass or fail a student in the clinical area may be ambiguous and inconsistent. It is important to note that many of the student factors that lead to a decision to fail a student, such as poor communication, unprofessional behavior, and being labeled as weak, are difficult to measure. They are also difficult to teach and faculty may assume that students should inherently know these behaviors.

It is important to think about your own experiences of receiving clinical evaluations, as these may affect how you evaluate students. Belinsky and Tataronis (2007) implemented a study ($n = 85$) to determine whether clinical instructors' previous experiences as radiation therapy students affected the process of how they currently evaluated students. Findings suggested that respondents who believed they had positive clinical experiences as students were more likely to have positive attitudes toward clinical evaluations of their current students. Thus, novice nurse educators may benefit from reflection on their own clinical experiences as students and how these may affect their approach to evaluation of their students.

The subtitle of this chapter—"Where Does Learning Stop and Evaluation Begin?"—suggests the difficulty of knowing when to decide whether to pass or fail a student. If a student is slow in learning content but conscientious, you want to ensure that you give him or her adequate time to master content and skills. However, a student who consistently fails to meet course objectives should not be passed on from course to course, only to be told before graduation that he or she is not performing satisfactorily. Thus, the nurse educator walks a difficult tightrope in the evaluation process.

If a faculty member does decide to fail a student, it can be a stressful process, especially for novice faculty. Educators may hesitate to document poor performance of a student because of the extensive documentation of the decision that may be required (Henderson & Eaton, 2013). Also, it may be difficult to seek advice from colleagues without betraying the confidentiality of the student. However, making a decision to fail a student is serious for both the student and you. As a new educator, you will benefit from advice of a colleague who can help you see how to best make this difficult decision. Often you can present the case to a colleague without betraying the confidentiality of the student.

STRATEGIES FOR EFFECTIVE CLINICAL EVALUATION

- Share clear expectations for students and obtain their individual goals for learning.
- Provide frequent opportunities for formative evaluation.
- Work collaboratively with nursing staff on the unit to ensure they are aware of your goals for the students.
- Consult with experienced educators to help you in difficult pass/fail decisions.
- Use clinical journals to provide opportunities for open dialogue between you and the student.
- Consider ways to use high- or low-fidelity simulation as a nonthreatening platform for practicing clinical skills and fostering self-reflection on performance.
- Use multiple sources for gathering data about student performance, such as observation, discussion with staff, and document review.

The National League for Nursing (NLN; 2005) Competency No. 3 calls for nurse educators to use a variety of strategies to assess and evaluate student learning in the cognitive, psychomotor, and affective domains and to provide timely, constructive, and thoughtful feedback to learners. To meet this competency, it is important to develop and implement evidence-based assessment and evaluation practices that are appropriate to the learner and learner goals.

Traditional approaches to evaluation of nursing students' performance focus on testing their acquisition of knowledge. Yet findings from the Carnegie Foundation for the Advancement of Teaching study suggested the need to move away from decontextualized knowledge and reframe assessment practices to focus on learning in real situations (Benner, Sutphen, Leonard, & Day, 2010). Poindexter, Hagler, and Lindell (2015) discussed the advantages of moving to an *authentic assessment*, in which students can demonstrate acquired knowledge, skills, and attitudes in a context of real-world nursing practice. This evaluation approach focuses not only on knowledge acquisition but also on assessment methods that test the ability to apply knowledge and integrate complex concepts.

More research is needed to provide evidence for student evaluation approaches that can be used not only to judge the competency of the student but also to enhance the teaching–learning process. In addition, faculty development programs for new nurse educators are needed to provide them with the necessary knowledge and skills to implement the evaluation process successfully (Johnson, 2014).

Questions for Reflection

1. The head nurse informs you angrily that John, one of your students on the orthopedic unit, has interfered with the traction set up on the bed. What would be your first action? What sort of further action would you consider?
2. Sarah has been on your clinical unit for 2 weeks and does not seem to be progressing. Faculty who have had her in other courses say that she is a "weak" student. What would your approach be for clinical evaluation of Sarah?
3. As you enter the clinical unit where your students will be coming later that day, you overhear two nurses talking about how unprofessional students are these days. What would you do?
4. Janice, a new graduate nurse who you think is performing competently on your clinical unit, asks to meet with you to discuss her performance. She tells you that she is very frustrated because she feels that she is not learning the skills that she should know. She is wondering if maybe nursing is not the right profession for her. How would you respond to Janice?

REFERENCES

Andrew, N. (2013). Clinical imprinting: The impact of early clinical learning on career long professional development in nursing. *Nurse Education in Practice, 13*(3), 161–164.

Belinsky, S. B., & Tataronis, G. R. (2007). Past experiences of the clinical instructor and current attitudes toward evaluation of students. *Journal of Allied Health, 36*(1), 11–16.

Benner, P., Sutphen, M., Leonard, V., & Day, L. (2010). *Educating nurses: A call for radical transformation*. San Francisco, CA: Jossey-Bass.

Cangelosi, P. R., Crocker, S., & Sorrell, J. M. (2009). Expert to novice: Clinicians learning new roles as clinical nurse educators. *Nursing Education Perspectives*, *30*, 367–371.

Cazzell, M., & Rodriguez, A. (2011). Qualitative analysis of student beliefs and attitudes after an objective structured clinical evaluation: Implications for affective domain learning in undergraduate nursing education. *Journal of Nursing Education*, *50*(12), 711–714.

DeBrew, J. K., & Lewallen, L. P. (2014). To pass or to fail? Understanding the factors considered by faculty in the clinical evaluation of nursing students. *Nurse Education Today*, *34*(4), 631–636.

Diekelmann, N., & McGregor, A. (2003). Students who fail clinical courses: Keeping open a future of new possibilities. *Journal of Nursing Education*, *42*(10), 433–436.

Duffy, K. (2013). Providing constructive feedback to students during mentoring. *Nursing Standard*, *27*(31), 50–56.

Heaslip, V., & Scammell, J. M. E. (2012). Failing underperforming students: The role of grading in practice assessment. *Nurse Education in Practice*, *12*(2), 95–100.

Henderson, A., & Eaton, E. (2013). Assisting nurses to facilitate student and new graduate learning in practice settings: What "support" do nurses at the bedside need? *Nurse Education in Practice*, *13*(3), 155–234.

Johnson, K. V. (2014). *Improving adjunct nursing instructors' knowledge of student assessment in clinical courses*. Doctoral dissertation. University of Arkansas. UMI Number: 3623189.

McCutchan, J. A. (2010). *The experience of baccalaureate degree seeking nursing students undergoing the process of clinical evaluation appraisal*. Doctoral dissertation. Indiana State University. UMI Number: 3404448.

National League for Nursing (NLN). (2005). *Core competencies of nurse educators*. Retrieved from http://www.nln.org/docs/default-source/default-document-library/core-competencies-of-nurse-educators-with-task-statements.pdf?sfvrsn=0

Plakht, Y., Shiyovich, A., Nusbaum, L., & Raizer, H. (2013). The association of positive and negative feedback with clinical performance, self-evaluation and practice contributions of nursing students. *Nurse Education Today*, *33*, 1261–1268.

Poindexter, K., Hagler, D., & Lindell, D. (2015). Designing authentic assessment. *Nurse Educator*, *40*(1), 36–40.

Rafiee, G., Moattari, M., Nikbakht, A. N., Kojuri, J., & Mousavinasab, M. (2014). Problems and challenges of nursing students' clinical evaluation: A qualitative study. *Iranian Journal of Nursing and Midwifery Research*, *19*(1), 41–49.

Zafrir, H., & Nissim, S. (2011). Evaluation in clinical practice using an innovation model for clinical teachers. *Journal of Nursing Education*, *50*(3), 167–171.

CHAPTER 5

Mentors Needed!

Please mentor me! Don't just orient me.

—Joanie

Nurse clinicians who have decided to transition to the clinical nurse educator role are usually enthusiastic and motivated to share their clinical expertise, but often have questions and anxieties about their transition from the clinical to the academic setting (Penn, Wilson, & Rosseter, 2008). Lack of self-confidence in a new role can lead to frustration and even a decision to resign from the position, creating increased costs for the institution, dissatisfaction for the nurses themselves, and lack of needed support for students. If expert clinicians are to be recruited and retained as educators, what are the best ways to help them become expert educators?

THE STORIES

One commonality noted in the literature that all faculty need, even crave, is mentoring (Cangelosi, Crocker, & Sorrell, 2009; Gardner, 2014; Siler & Kleiner, 2001; Smith & Zsohar, 2007). Nurses who are learning the clinical nurse educator role not only need preceptors to help them understand the "how to" role aspects to achieve competencies, but also they need mentors to help them understand the context and big picture of the role. Participants in the Clinical Nurse Educator Academy shared their reflections of what they believed was needed in their new role (Cangelosi et al., 2009). They responded to the following prompt:

> Think about the role of mentoring in nursing. Describe an incident that reflects your ideas about what you need from a mentor as you move to a new role as clinical nurse educator.

As Joanie, a participant in the academy, exclaimed in the quote at the start of this chapter, mentoring is a key requirement that novice faculty need. "Fear," "pain," and "frustration" were palpable in the narratives of these new nurse educators. Many feared not being able to teach effectively, despite their clinical expertise. How does one transfer this clinical knowledge to a nursing student? Pain and frustration were experienced when the novice educator realized how "out of my comfort zone I am." For years, these nurses honed clinical skills and now felt competent and in control in a clinical setting; yet, when faced with students, these same nurses suddenly felt incompetent to transfer their vast clinical knowledge to help students learn.

Orientation Versus Mentoring

Orientation is essential. Clinical hours, planning a clinical day, evaluating students, knowing where to park, how to get security badges, and all of the minutiae that is embedded in clinical teaching are critical for the novice clinical faculty member to learn, and are appropriate topics for orientation programs. Classroom orientation helps, but only goes so far. It is very scary for a novice educator to be "alone" in a clinical agency and face not only clinical questions, but student issues and time management concerns, as well. Mentoring was voiced as key in the successful adjustment to the educator role. To some, orientation may equal mentoring. However, as Joanie clearly stated, there is a difference between mentoring and orientation:

As I seriously, yet cautiously, consider becoming a clinical nurse educator, I realize that there will be a multitude of skills, competencies, and educational-related "tasks" that I will have to master. Some components of clinical teaching will be easier to learn than others.... There will be many (I pray) who will step up to the plate and orient me. These folks will tell me how to keep accurate records, where to submit grades, how to contact clinical site coordinators, where to make copies of hand-outs, and so on. They will answer my questions and make sure that I follow policies and procedures so that I am compliant with the ways of the teaching world. Those that orient me will play an integral part in my success as a new clinical educator and I will greatly appreciate their efforts. However, I know that I will want (and need) ongoing support, encouragement, and expert guidance along my career journey. I will surely need a mentor.

A mentor will not be "assigned" to me. I will seek out someone whom I trust, respect, and who has expertise in the clinical education arena. Ideally, this person will also choose me, and a collaborative working and social relationship will ensue. I want my mentor to back me up when I'm right and offer constructive criticism when I'm wrong and "way off base." I need this person to be brutally honest with me when I veer from my set goals, so that I can continue to improve and grow positively in my profession. I also would like this person to feel so inclined to hug me when I'm ready to "throw in the towel" or laugh with me over my silly mistakes. As an added bonus, I would like this person to become a lifelong friend.

One novice clinical educator confided:

I get so sidetracked. There is so much going on, so many student needs I have to tend to, and so much I have to remember—not to mention the patient issues. I don't know how to organize all of it, and some days—no, most days— I just want to quit. I feel so out of sorts! And you know what makes me feel the worst? I am not a good role model for the students like this.

Orientation is a distant memory for a novice educator who is feeling overwhelmed. "Alone" in the clinical setting, orientation knowledge is quickly overlooked or even forgotten. What these novice educators desperately need is mentoring.

Preceptor Versus Mentor

If they are fortunate, new nurse educators may be assigned a preceptor who will help them become comfortable with the day-to-day activities that they need to know. This kind of supervision is helpful, but it does not equate to the mentor role. Rose shared how she saw the preceptor role and mentor role differently:

> The role of mentoring is crucial in nurse success. While most of us have worked with or as preceptors, the role of a mentor differs, in that it imposes less structure and is a fluid role, versus guidance over a set period of time. While many hospitals, such as my own, have implemented formal mentoring programs, I feel that the role of a mentor is one that develops through a process. Sometimes the best mentors are not those who we have defined as a resource person or expert, but someone who provides us guidance and support and understands our current situation.
>
> Such is the role of a mentor—to challenge the novice to adapt the skills and critical thinking needed to succeed in a new role.
>
> Although I am just beginning my journey into the clinical nurse educator role, I am in need of a mentor who will both guide me along my education and transition me into a teaching role…ease me into this new role, appreciate my talents and [the] abilities I bring with me, and challenge me to work hard. I function best under someone who is strict, pushes me to my limit, but gives me positive feedback when I have succeeded. For me, a mentor does not do the work for me, but shows me how to do it, employs creative ways to pass along knowledge, and takes the time to hear my frustrations, complaints, or achievements. Because a mentor is a less defined role than a preceptor, I feel this

person can also serve as a friend and should feel that they can gain from my knowledge and skill as well.

Frances clearly expressed her need for a mentor even though she had already had some previous teaching experience:

> Now that I am embarking on the educator role, I know that I will be a novice and that there will be a new learning curve to gain expertise in the education arena. My biggest concern is not having a mentor in place for me, to help me learn and grow from discussions and feedback. There is a definite fear of being incompetent and not doing a good job even though I teach formally and informally in my occupation now.

Ellyn provided a detailed description of the different types of support that a preceptor and mentor provided for her:

> Studies have shown that effective mentoring can make the difference between students' and novice nurses' decision to stay in nursing and find fulfillment, or become disillusioned and leave the profession.
>
> Thus was the case for me when as a student I was hired 30 years ago as a full-time summer patient care technician during my senior year in nursing school. The staff nurse that was assigned to orient me, a relatively new nurse herself, showed me what to do during patient care assignments and after 2 weeks I was basically left to my own devices. Externally I looked like I was doing alright, but inside I was terrified and I was acutely anxious that I would make a mistake. After 4 weeks, the nurse that was supposed to supervise me co-signed my charts without actually observing my work. Soon I found myself giving medications, including IV meds and narcotics, changing dressings, and giving multiple patient treatments. Despite the fact that I seemed to be able to handle assignments, inside I was totally overwhelmed and seriously doubted that I could do this kind of work as a career. No one noticed my insecurities except for Sara, the head nurse who became my informal mentor. Besides her busy schedule,

she took me under her wings and showed me the caring aspect of patient care. From her example, I learned how important it is to truly connect with patients. She took her time listening to their concerns.... She also took the time to listen to my fears and concerns. When she discovered how insecure I actually was about my nursing care ability, she made sure to be there for me as a resource and support.

I learned from her also the importance of team work and camaraderie. She set the example by answering call lights whenever available, following through with whatever the patient requested or needed. Her role modeling enabled me to increase my confidence—not only in my ability to care for patients, but also in how to prioritize care. I sought her out whenever I could and she always took the time to teach me skills I wanted to master, as well as teach me rationale behind nursing practice. I never forget how she let me start IVs in her arm, despite that fact that it took several attempts. By the time I finished nursing school and passed my boards, I had discovered the "joy of nursing" and continued working at the same institution.

The lessons I learned from Sara's mentoring have stayed with me throughout my nursing career.... Mentoring should not be seen as a duty, but as a work of love to train the next generation of competent and caring clinical nurses.

What Constitutes Mentoring in Nursing?

What does a mentor in nursing need to know or do? How does one learn to be a mentor? Conversations with nurses have revealed that there is not a consistent understanding of what constitutes mentoring in nursing and there is little formal preparation for this role. It is interesting that Jill can remember various mentors in different phases of her life, but not in her clinical experiences:

I have to honestly say that I have had some incredible role models in my life. Many of whom were nursing instructors and professors. On the other hand, I can't really think of any mentors that I have had in my clinical life....

I know I need a mentor who truly respects me. I need a mentor who encourages me. I need a mentor who serves as my role model. One who affirms that what I do is meaningful, effective, and valid. I need a mentor who helps me to help myself.

Sabrina emphasized the importance for a mentor to listen and be nonjudgmental and honest when interacting with students:

I think that mentors need to approach students with a positive attitude and be strength-based, though that doesn't mean pretending everything is wonderful if it isn't. It's also important to be honest with students in a way that is sensitive to the situation and their feelings....

It's also helpful when mentors are good listeners. If you listen well to students, you will be much more aware of what their needs are and how to support them. Mentors need to individualize their approach to their students and recognize each student's needs and strengths.

I think it's also important that mentors not micromanage their students. Students need to understand what's expected of them, and then be allowed to fulfill those expectations without an instructor watching every move they make. However, mentors need to be readily available to students not only in terms of a physical presence, but also in terms of being a resource to the students.

When I think of those people in my life who have been mentors to me, I also see intelligence and integrity as important traits. Respecting what the mentor has to say is kind of an essential starting point. If a student doesn't have an interest in the mentor to begin with, then none of the rest matters. Basically, good mentoring means being able to *connect* with students, so skills, such as good listening, being strength-based, and so on, will facilitate those "connections." Also a good mentor should *show the way* in terms of how they negotiate the role you are trying to adopt, so skills such as integrity, intelligence, etc., will help in creating paths for students.

Jennie added characteristics of a mentor that are important to her:

> Using the theory of "expert to novice" I will need my
> mentor to understand that I was an expert in my old
> role as a clinician, but a novice in my new role as a clini-
> cal nurse… and I will need from her some guidance
> and instructions. I will need my mentor to offer me help
> when I need help, and to see both of us as a team work-
> ing toward a common goal of pursuing continuous
> quality improvement in our nurse educator role. When
> I encounter difficulty or frustration in my new role, I will
> need my mentor to be able to encourage and give me the
> support that I need to function effectively. I will need
> my mentor to be able to give me advice on how to solve
> problems in difficult situations.… I will expect positive
> and negative feedback. I will use feedback gained from
> self, peers, and mentor to improve my role effectiveness.
> I will need my mentor to recognize the five stage model
> of skill acquisition of novice, advanced beginner, compe-
> tent, proficient, and expert. Recognizing these five stages
> will help my mentor to meet my needs along these five
> stages. In addition, I will need my mentor to respect me
> as an adult learner, and that we all have different learn-
> ing styles. I will also expect my mentor and me to have
> a good interpersonal relationship. According to the lec-
> ture on creating positive clinical learning experiences for
> students, interpersonal relationships were viewed as the
> most highly valued characteristics rated by both students
> and clinical educators. In conclusion, as I move to a role
> of a nurse educator, I need a mentor who can give guid-
> ance and support, who has the ability to create an envi-
> ronment conducive to learning, who can serve as a role
> model and communicate effectively.

Chapter 1 included a story from Veronica, in which she described how discouraged she felt as a novice educator and getting "fired" by her preceptor. Here, she continues her story to describe how important it was for her to have a mentor during the period of time that she was gaining experience and confidence in the nurse educator role:

Where had I gone wrong? I reviewed the last 2 months, examined our interactions, and began to see the cracks. I had been overly demanding. I had pushed Lorna too hard. I had tried new ways of teaching, but they weren't what she had needed. Crumbled and despairing, I went to the one person I knew who could help me: Sally.

Sally was like me, fast-forwarded 30 years. Sally was dreaming of a career in nursing education, and she was in a master's program. She had been a labor and delivery nurse for 30 years, and she had a passion for teaching new hires. I considered Sally my mother-figure on the unit, the gentle embrace I could go to for a listening ear, a guiding hand, and a warm hug. Sally was my mentor.

I took Sally aside on the unit, during a particularly quiet day. I told her everything: the call, the devastation, the fallout. She took me into an empty labor room, and she hugged me. Then she looked into my eyes, and she said something that would stay with me for years to come: "Veronica, you know, even though you're a teacher, you still have to learn how to teach." I was startled, and I didn't entirely understand what she meant, at first. She went on, "Nobody knows how to teach when they first begin. And, yeah, this time didn't work out. You probably did push Lorna too hard. You know, you always have to keep in mind your student when you're teaching. You have to adjust your methods to the person. But, you know, this was your first time teaching. Don't get down about it. Learn from it. You'll do better next time."

I looked at her, questioning. "Maybe there shouldn't be a next time. Maybe I'm just not cut out for this." Sally smiled. "Of course you are. You can't let this one time get you down. You're gonna be a great teacher some day. But, you just have to learn from this. Get through this experience, and learn from it."

"But, Sally, what about everybody else? What about the other nurses? I mean, I know they know what happened. I just, I just feel so stupid!" "Don't worry about it!" Sally assured me. "They may know, but they don't really care. Don't let it get to you."

So with a hug, Sally sent me off, shaken, but stirred on to a new start. I absorbed all of what had just happened, and I processed what it all meant to me. Suddenly, I felt rejuvenated—and free. I didn't have to be the Perfect Teacher. I could make mistakes. And moreover, I could make those mistakes in front of everyone, and it would still be okay. They would forget, but I would carry with me valuable lessons for the future. I realized how much I needed Sally, my mentor; how I couldn't be confident and strong all the time; and how even—no, *especially*— teachers need a little guidance every now and then. I would finish orienting Lorna and many other students in the future, but I didn't have to do it alone. After all, teachers need each other, so they can keep on teaching—and learning.

Veronica's story makes one think that she may be in a very different point in her career today if she had not had Sally as a mentor.

REFLECTIONS FOR NEW NURSE EDUCATORS

The nursing literature includes helpful information for orientation of full-time nurse educators who are new to a particular nursing program. In a mentoring needs assessment implemented by Sawatzky and Enns (2009), researchers found that the most significant stressor for novice faculty was "fitting in" to the academic culture. Cangelosi (2004) and Suplee and Gardner (2009) described carefully planned and programmed faculty development programs for new full-time faculty at their respective universities. Research development is emphasized in some mentoring programs (Records & Emerson, 2003) while a number of new faculty actually mentor themselves in the role of faculty scholar (Jacelon, Zucker, Staccarine, & Henneman, 2003; Lewallen, Crane, Letvak, Jones, & Hu, 2003). General tips and strategies for novice faculty on how to lead an academic life are also included in the literature (Bellack, 2003; Mann, 2004).

Although many nursing programs provide mentors for new full-time educators to help them learn the role of the nurse educator (Culleiton & Shellenbarger, 2007), neophyte part-time clinical faculty also require specialized orientation. Part-time faculty have some unique needs that must be addressed, such as keeping abreast of what the students are learning in the classroom and how this affects the students' clinical instruction. Despite the fact that health care disciplines recognize that mentoring programs are needed for part-time faculty (Hewitt & Lewallen, 2010; Notzer & Abramovitz, 2008; O'Callaghan, 2007), there is little noted in the nursing literature that addresses this topic. In addition, there is a dearth of literature in nursing describing the preparation of mentors. Programs addressing the education of mentors in various disciplines are discussed in the literature (Gagen & Bowie, 2005; Pfund, Pribbenow, Branchaw, Lauffer, & Handelsman, 2006), but there is a need for a focus on preparation of nursing mentors. If nurse educators are considered to be experts, it seems to be assumed that they can also be expert mentors for new faculty members. Unfortunately, as Veronica has shown, this is not always true.

The Mentoring Relationship

Mentoring is both a concept and a relationship that must be embraced, encouraged, and fostered in the culture of nursing education. A mentoring relationship can be for the short or long term and can be tailored to meet the needs of each new educator. For the short term, a mentor is needed who is skilled in the policies of the university, the courses the novice faculty member is teaching, and teaching–learning principles. Long-term mentoring usually involves research and scholarship components, which would require a mentor proficient in these areas.

It is not unusual to have more than one mentor because it is difficult for one person to acquire all the skills new nurse educators require. As with nurse clinicians, nurse educators come with a variety of education skill sets. Philosophies of teaching may be well formulated or nonexistent, and knowledge of the teaching and evaluation processes may be evident, but not in agreement with the student who will be mentored. In addition, some novice nurse educators may be more adventurous, have a higher tolerance for uncertainty, and deal more constructively with the gray areas of the teaching and learning process. In these and many other instances, a skilled mentor can help the new faculty member adapt, learn, and thrive in the new environment.

Unfortunately, a new faculty member is often hired to replace the only person who would be the best mentor, making finding an appropriate and effective mentor(s) even more difficult (Gagen & Bowie, 2005). In orientation sessions, mentors may be assigned to new faculty; however, new faculty may seek out other mentors who fill other needs and who may be a better fit in personality, clinical and/or teaching expertise, and mentoring skill (McDonald, 2010). The goal of any orientation program as far as mentorship should be the provision of the initial mentorship structure early in the new faculty member's employment with the allowance for the evolution of this and other mentoring relationships (Suplee & Gardner, 2009).

Effective mentoring requires a significant time commitment on the part of the mentor. The mentor needs to be available to the mentee on a regular basis, meet regularly with the mentee, and even make clinical site visits if necessary. This is a real challenge in light of the current nursing faculty shortage and the high demands placed on full-time faculty. Mentors also need to have a genuine interest in the concerns and the success of their mentees. The new faculty member can sense when he or she is viewed as insignificant, a nuisance, or a drain on the faculty member's time and resources.

Mentoring must be supported by administration and factored into the faculty member's workload; otherwise, it will not receive the attention it both deserves and requires. Hiring experienced part-time faculty to ease the full-time faculty member's load while mentoring would be an investment that would pay off in huge dividends if the novice educator obtained excellent mentoring and became an expert nurse educator (Cangelosi, 2014). Effective mentoring relationships have been linked to more effective teaching, possible increased productivity, and a smoother transition and increased retention of new educators (Billings & Kowalski, 2008; White, Brannan, & Wilson, 2010; Wilson, Brannan, & White, 2010). As McDonald (2010, p. 131) claims, "A mentor may mean the difference between retention and exodus from the academic setting."

As identified in National League for Nursing (NLN) Core Competency No. 6, it is the responsibility of nurse educators to "Pursue Continuous Quality Improvement in the Nurse Educator Role," an important element of which is "mentors and supports faculty colleagues" (NLN, 2005). Given the tremendous responsibilities and time commitments of nurse educators today, it is difficult to find time and resources to implement effective mentorship programs, either in a school of nursing or hospital. Yet, it is essential that this need be addressed. Novice nurse educators need mentoring in all of the NLN Core Competencies in order to be effective in their role.

Perhaps Estelle, an expert nurse clinician and novice educator in the Clinical Nurse Educator Academy, summed up the importance of mentoring best when she said,

> If we provide an enabling environment, then it is my strong belief that novice educators will blossom and will be great assets for that school. If a university wants excellence from their teachers, then university faculty have to spend time and find out what novice teachers need and work on it. We cannot use trial and error theory with our new faculty and students, because, chances are, it can fail both of them.

Strategies for Successful Mentoring Relationships

- Identify what you want and need in a mentor.
- Seek out one or more persons who can mentor you. Share with them what you need from them.
- Your mentor does not need to be a nurse. Sometimes there are friends or colleagues in other disciplines who may be very effective mentors for you.
- Make the mentoring relationship a win–win experience for both you and your mentor. Think about how you can make the relationship with your mentor beneficial for him or her, as well as you.
- Keep a reflective journal that describes your mentoring experiences and share these with your mentor.

Questions for Reflection

1. You accept a part-time position as a nurse educator while still working at your clinical job, but no mentor is assigned to help you adjust to your new role. How would you go about finding a suitable mentor?
2. A friend asks you what you would want in a mentor. What would you say?

3. Think back on a time when someone mentored you. What did they do that made a difference for you?

4. As a new educator in your school of nursing, you are asked to identify what should be included in a mentorship program. What important elements should be included?

5. You believe that your hospital should implement a mentoring program for new nurse graduates, but you know that the budget will not allow hiring of new personnel to serve as mentors. What creative options could you suggest for implementing a mentoring program?

REFERENCES

Bellack, J. P. (2003). Advice for new (and seasoned) faculty. *Journal of Nursing Education, 42,* 383–384.

Billings, D., & Kowalski, K. (2008). Developing your career as a nurse educator: The importance of having (or being) a mentor. *The Journal of Continuing Education in Nursing, 39,* 490–491.

Cangelosi, P. R. (2004). A lack of qualified faculty: One school's solution. *Nurse Educator, 29,* 186–188.

Cangelosi, P. R. (2014). Novice nurse faculty: In search of a mentor. *Nursing Education Perspectives, 35,* 327–329.

Cangelosi, P. R., Crocker, S., & Sorrell, J. M. (2009). Expert to novice: Clinicians learning new roles as clinical nurse educators. *Nursing Education Perspectives, 30,* 367–371.

Culleiton, A. L., & Shellenbarger, T. (2007). Transition of a bedside clinician to a nurse educator. *MEDSURG Nursing, 16,* 253–257.

Gagen, L., & Bowie, S. (2005). Effective mentoring: A case for training mentors for novice teachers. *Journal of Physical Education, Recreation, & Dance, 76*(7), 40–45.

Gardner, S. S. (2014). From learning to teach to teaching effectiveness: Nurse educators describe their experiences. *Nursing Education Perspectives, 35,* 106–111.

Hewitt, P., & Lewallen, L. P. (2010). Ready, set, teach! How to transform the clinical nurse expert into the part-time clinical nurse instructor. *Journal of Continuing Education in Nursing, 41,* 403–407.

Jacelon, C. S., Zucker, D. M., Staccarine, J., & Henneman, E. A. (2003). Peer mentoring for tenure-track faculty. *Journal of Professional Nursing, 19,* 335–338.

Lewallen, L. P., Crane, P. B., Letbak, S., Jones, E., & Hu, J. (2003). An innovative strategy to enhance new faculty success. *Nursing Education Perspectives, 24,* 257–260.

Mann, A. S. (2004). Eleven tips for the new college teacher. *Journal of Nursing Education, 43,* 389–390.

McDonald, P. J. (2010). Transitioning from clinical practice to nursing faculty: Lessons learned. *Journal of Nursing Education, 49,* 126–131.

National League for Nursing. (2005). Core competencies of nurse educators with task statements. Retrieved from http://www.nln.org/profdev/core-competencies.pdf

Notzer, N., & Abramovitz, R. (2008). Can brief workshops improve clinical instruction? *Medical Education, 42,* 152–156.

O'Callaghan, N. (2007). Addressing clinical preceptor teaching development. *The Journal of Physician Assistant Education, 18*(4), 37–39.

Penn, B. K., Wilson, L. D., & Rosseter, R. (2008, Sept.) Transitioning from nursing practice to a teaching role. *Online Journal of Issues in Nursing, 13*(3), Manuscript 3.

Pfund, C., Pribbenow, C. M., Branchaw, J., Lauffer, S. M., & Handelsman, J. (2006). The merits of training mentors. *Science, 311,* 473–474.

Records, K., & Emerson, R. J. (2003). Mentoring for research skill development. *Journal of Nursing Education, 42,* 553–557.

Sawatzky, J., & Enns, C. L. (2009). A mentoring needs assessment: Validating mentorship in nursing education. *Journal of Professional Nursing, 25,* 145–150.

Siler, B. B., & Kleiner, C. (2001). Novice faculty: Encountering expectations in academia. *Journal of Nursing Education, 40,* 397–403.

Smith, J. A., & Zsohar, H. (2007). Essentials of neophyte mentorship in relation to the faculty shortage. *Journal of Nursing Education, 46,* 184–186.

Suplee, P. D., & Gardner, M. (2009). Fostering a smooth transition to the faculty role. *The Journal of Continuing Education in Nursing, 40,* 514–520.

White, A., Brannan, J., & Wilson, C. B. (2010). A mentor–protégé program for new faculty, Part I: Stories of protégés. *Journal of Nursing Education, 49*(11), 601–607.

Wilson, C. B., Brannan, J., & White, A. (2010). A mentor—protégé program for new faculty, Part II: Stories of mentors. *Journal of Nursing Education, 49*(12), 665–671.

Teaching Thinking

CHAPTER 6

Socratic Pedagogy: Teaching Students to Think Like Nurses

Christine Sorrell Dinkins

Education isn't what some people declare it to be, namely, putting knowledge into souls that lack it, like putting sight into blind eyes. But our present discussion, on the other hand, shows that the power to learn is present in everyone's soul and that the instrument with which each learns is like an eye that cannot be turned around from darkness to light without turning the whole body.

—Socrates (Plato, 518c, trans. 1992c)

Through the years since nursing education has moved from hospitals into colleges and universities, what nurses need to learn and know has changed dramatically. What has not changed substantially is the way students are taught to learn and know. One of the major recommendations from the study sponsored by the Carnegie Foundation for the Advancement of Teaching, *Educating Nurses: A Call for Radical Transformation,* was the need to "Expand the focus on critical thinking to an emphasis on clinical reasoning and multiple ways of thinking" (Benner, Sutphen, Leonard, & Day, 2010, p. 89). Thus, this chapter introduces a new approach to teaching thinking, Socratic pedagogy. Clinical nurse educators can use Socratic pedagogy to bridge the knowledge–action gap that students and new graduate nurses often experience by helping each of them learn to think like a nurse.

One question to ask about this chapter might be, "What is a philosophy professor doing writing a chapter in a book for nurse educators?" Philosophy has a strong and proud connection with nursing and nursing education, thanks to Patricia Benner, Nancy Diekelmann, Jean Watson, and others who brought to nursing an attention to phenomenology, hermeneutics, and other philosophical ways of thinking and knowing. In addition, philosophy happens to be the home discipline for many of the oldest and best explorations of education—from Parmenides in 6th century BCE to John Dewey in the 20th century. In between those two, of course, in the 5th century BCE, was perhaps the most famous teacher of all, Socrates.

We know a little about the historical Socrates—he was a teacher before all else in his life, he was devoted to his students and to his beloved city of Athens, and he was tried, convicted, and executed for corrupting the youth. Since Socrates never wrote anything, we know him best through the writings of his greatest student, Plato. Nearly all of Plato's works are constructed dialogues featuring Socrates as the main character. How close is this character to the historical Socrates? That is a matter of debate. But regardless of historical authenticity, the character of Socrates in Plato's works is a model teacher. Looking into his comportment and the methods he used to lead his students in inquiry, readers today can gain great insights into new (but very old!) ways of teaching.

"Socratic pedagogy" is not a consistently defined term, and in fact it is a term often misused (Kost & Chen, 2015). In this chapter, this term refers to a philosophy of teaching based on the model of Socrates in Plato's dialogues. It is a type of teaching that requires active learning and engagement from students and teacher alike, and thus is particularly valuable for teaching in the clinical area. Throughout the chapter, illustrations from Plato's works serve as explanations of Socrates's teaching philosophy and as models for clinical nurse educators to follow.

WHY SOCRATIC PEDAGOGY?

New Teaching Methods Are Needed

Nursing education is a complex challenge for even the most experienced nurse educators. Nursing students and newly hired nurses must learn a tremendous volume of knowledge, skills, critical thinking, and ethical reasoning, and must know how to put all these resources together in their care for patients. In this era when new information, theories, and facts are being produced at a rapid pace, "nurse educators are faced with the need to do more than help students recall facts ... they are challenged to assist students to learn how to learn for a lifetime" (Rogge, 2001, p. 69). Students need to know how to apply and synthesize what they have learned in the classroom, but they also need to know how to continue learning, processing, and synthesizing new information throughout their careers.

In addition to teaching in such a challenging era, educators may have trouble developing new pedagogies and active teaching strategies because of "lack of time, student and faculty resistance, structural barriers, and the academy's devaluing of the scholarship of teaching" (Tedesco-Schneck, 2013, p. 59). Thus, the Carnegie Foundation study on nursing education (Benner et al., 2010) was a much-needed call to action, a call to give nurse educators the resources and support they need to develop the unique teaching skills required for educating within a practice. The report found that students receive little education on setting priorities, even though this skill is critical for providing safe patient care. The report also found that students are often asked to learn from lectures and linear PowerPoint presentations, but students find they tune out or lose focus when learning using these formats. In addition, the report identified a need for teaching everyday ethics, as opposed to artificial dilemmas taught in ethical theory classes, and a need to teach skills for reflective practice. As Marlow et al. (2015) state, "the concern is on moving away from a content-driven didactic teaching to a learning environment that is dialogic, open, allows for multiple perspectives, and creates space to challenge assumptions and to develop a sense of ethical knowing" (p. 26).

A call for teaching thinking in nursing education is not new, and in fact Benner is concerned that "critical thinking" has become more of a catch-all phrase for how teachers want students to think, rather than a focus on teaching specific ways of learning and knowing that nurses need for competent practice (Benner et al., 2010). Benner, Hughes, and Sutphen (2008) emphasize that while "critical reflective skills are essential for clinicians," nurses' thinking must include much more: "reflection, induction, deduction, analysis, challenging assumptions, and evaluation of data and information to guide decision-making." To educate nurses for these diverse skills, Benner et al. (2010) recommend a movement away from a simple emphasis on critical thinking to an emphasis on multiple ways of thinking, including "the ability to reason as a clinical situation changes, taking into account the context and concerns of the patient and family ... as well as critical, creative and scientific reasoning" (p. 85).

Socratic Pedagogy Helps Students Develop Critical Thinking and Other Key Skills

Nurse educators are faced with the stress of covering more and more information in their teaching as new evidence for best practices in caring for patients evolves from research. Yet, considering that "covering" something also means to obscure it, one realizes that even if it were possible to give students all the essential information needed in their practice, it would be counter-productive to try to do so. Thus, nurse educators need teaching approaches to help students develop thinking skills that will encourage continued learning. Socratic dialogue— a question-driven, student-centered, discussion-based shared inquiry between teachers and students—builds confidence and reliability in students by helping them think through why they do what they do: why they make certain decisions, why they look at certain situations in a particular way. In Plato's dialogues, Socrates explains that beliefs and opinions need to be "tied down" so that they do not run away or lead us to error. The more we can justify our beliefs by pondering our reasons for holding them and also the connections between the beliefs, the more reliable and high-quality our decisions will be (Plato, 97d, trans. 1981d).

Socratic pedagogy is not about asking questions with specific answers in mind; it is an active engagement in dialogue, asking students to think and be creative in their answers, while the instructor remains open to what the students might respond or ask. And it is not just about giving feedback on a particular situation or recently completed task, it is about helping students learn to think and to apply the learning from the current moment to situations in the future. Engaging students in dialogue helps them connect the dots between what they learned in pathophysiology or pharmacology class and what is happening here, now with their patients.

In Plato's dialogue *Meno* (trans. 1981d), Socrates offers an image to help explain why beliefs and opinions need to be examined and justified in order to become reliable knowledge. He evokes the statues of

Daedalus, which were reportedly so lifelike they would run away if not tied down. Like these statues, Socrates explains, even true and accurate beliefs "run away and escape if one does not tie them down" (97d). In a similar explanation in the *Republic* (Plato, trans. 1992c), Socrates asks, "do you think that those who express a true opinion without knowledge or understanding are any different from blind people who happen to travel the right road?" (506c). For Socrates, if we make decisions based on untested opinions or on facts we have not considered and contextualized, we are operating in the darkness; these opinions and facts may help us find the right path, but we cannot reliably stick to that path, partly because we do not know *why* it is the right path.

Throughout Plato's dialogues, the distinction Socrates and his dialogue partners (usually referred to as his interlocutors) consistently make is that true beliefs and genuine knowledge will point to the same direction, but true belief cannot be trusted to stay with a person. A nursing student who has learned the course content or a particular skill may do well when situations are typical, relaxed, or straightforward, but the student will be more likely to make an error if the situation is more complicated or he or she is under time pressure. Once that student has examined and "tied down" his or her course content and skills, that is, once the student has knowledge and understanding, he or she will more reliably know, and be able to follow through on, the right decision in a complicated situation.

The beauty of teaching through dialogue and employing Socratic pedagogy is that it gives educators the opportunity to address skills called for in recent reports and articles on the future of nursing education: ethical thinking, creative thinking, learning to learn, and adapting to rapidly changing situations. Moreover, since Socratic pedagogy is student-centered, it tends to keep students engaged more than lecture alone, allowing them to be active participants in their own learning. Socratic pedagogy allows the instructor to respond to the needs of the moment and of the student, so that students learn what they need to know *when* they need to know it, leading to better retention and comprehension. Imagine a clinical post conference that was originally intended to stick to the objective for the day, "end-of-life care," but a student raises an ethical question, or makes a statement that the instructor believes points to an ethical problem, such as assisted suicide. The instructor can then follow on that change of the conversation, taking that student and his or her peers down a path of inquiry that responds to the moment and the situation.

Benner et al. (2008) argue that "critical reflection requires that the thinker examine the underlying assumptions and radically question or doubt the validity of arguments, assertions, and even facts of the case." Socratic questioning does just that—it seeks out and exposes false assumptions and gaps in knowledge. By comparing beliefs and assumptions of one student or several, the questioning "focuses on one's desire not to contradict oneself and thus allows the teacher to compel the student to examine her or his internal incoherences" (Bloch-Schulman, 2012, p. 20).

Some educators may be concerned that Socratic teaching is less efficient than lecture, since discussion will always take more time than would the teacher simply speaking to the students, formally or informally. However, Garlikov (n.d.) notes that Socratic dialogue is "a very efficient teaching method, because the first time through tends to cover the topic very thoroughly, in terms of their understanding it." Even though a teacher can always lecture in less time, this method "gives constant feedback and thus allows monitoring of the students' understanding as you go. So you know what problems and misunderstandings or lack of understandings you need to address as you are presenting the material" (Garlikov, n.d.). In a clinical setting, this means instructors can structure a pre-conference to review the patients who are assigned to the students that day, and by asking questions and engaging in dialogue with the students, guide them to think about what to notice in their patients, what they can expect will happen, and catch any problems, misunderstandings, or false assumptions sooner and more efficiently than without dialogue.

Since the dialogue will almost always happen in a group, not only does this method help individual students analyze their own decisions and learn from any mistakes or misunderstandings, but peers will also learn from hearing these conversations or from joining them. As Boghossian (2003) points out, "Socratic pedagogy impacts the entire learning community because even those students who are hesitant to speak up … can benefit from seeing a genuine discourse modeled" (p. 20). Just as the historical Socrates taught and learned with his students gathered together, dialogue in today's teaching settings nearly always has an audience or a group to join in, and that larger group benefits from the experience nearly as much as those engaged directly in the conversation.

Socratic pedagogy asks the teacher to be a member of a community of learning with his or her students. The pedagogy is student-centered in that student needs and responses drive the inquiry, but the teacher remains an important guide at all times. Such a pedagogy helps create "a community of scholars because it requires the teacher to take seriously what students think and say and it encourages teacher and students to rely on each other for learning" (Rogge, 2001, p. 68). In a Socratic exchange in a simulation lab or a classroom, "assumptions and beliefs are challenged, questioned, and discussed communally in the moment. It is through this communal process of being actively engaged with one another and the subject matter at hand that new understandings arise" (Marlow et al., 2015, p. 26). As a group, students participating in Socratic pedagogy have many opportunities for ethical thinking and creative thinking as they discuss with their teacher and each other their thoughts and concerns about what they have learned or things they have done in patient care that day. And in that process of discussion, they are always learning to learn, developing a habit of questioning, analyzing, reflecting, and comparing ideas with their peers and supervisors. Such a habit serves them well as they head into a career where they must often adapt to rapidly changing situations.

Socratic Pedagogy Can Be Used in Many Educational Settings

Socratic pedagogy is as much a matter of comportment and student-centered focus as it is questioning and dialogue. Therefore, Socratic pedagogy can result in long, complex, sweeping discussions or small, quiet moments of exchange. Socratic questioning works very well during clinical conference or in a brief conversation in a hallway after seeing a patient. It can happen one-on-one between teacher and student, or as a discussion among a group, or with a group listening to a one-on-one conversation. A Socratic discussion in a clinical conference might go something like this:

Teacher: Luisa, tell us about the patient you cared for today.

Luisa: Well, he has X illness and is struggling with Y. He wasn't feeling very well today.

Teacher: What is your understanding of X illness? Luisa? Others? [Students give responses.]

Teacher: John, I notice you included the detail of "ABCD" when others did not. Do you think that detail is important here?

John: Yes.

Teacher: Why? Can you explain your reasoning to us?

John: Uh ...

Teacher: [laughs gently] Can someone help John out? Why might this detail be important?

(The conversation would then continue, with the teacher helping to guide the students in inquiry about this patient or other patients they saw on the unit that day.)

Socratic pedagogy serves well whenever an instructor wants to help students make connections between things—vital signs, the patient's current behavior, the baseline, a patient's previous behavior. The Socratic method is designed to connect beliefs and break ideas and questions down into component parts, ideal for teaching in a practice setting such as nursing. If a student in a simulation lab suggests, "I think we should try X" the teacher can ask, "Well, what would X do?" The student may respond that it would accomplish Y result. The teacher might then ask, "What might be higher priority than Y?" or "What might be more effective than X?" The teacher could then open the discussion up to other students: "Do you agree? Why or why not?" Or, if a student is feeling overwhelmed with data or options, a teacher can help him or her focus. "What data do you have? What have you observed? What do *you* think you need to focus on within all that data? Why?" If the student indicates focusing on A or B, the teacher can ask, "And how do those connect to C? Is C important here?"

THE SOCRATIC APPROACH: TEACHING AS AN ACT OF CARING

Common Misconceptions About Socratic Pedagogy

Socratic questioning and Socratic pedagogy in general should always grow out of respect and care for students. Too often in portrayals in popular media—or in practice in some education—Socratic questioning involves embarrassing students and calling them out, trying to catch them in a mistake or expose gaps in their knowledge. The fact is that Socratic questioning is *excellent* for catching students' gaps and mistakes, but it can be done in a respectful and caring way that allows all present to benefit from dialogue, especially the student being questioned (Kost & Chen, 2015). The questioning should not be antagonistic—a little uncomfortable or slightly anxiety-producing, perhaps, but always with the understanding that the dialogue is expressly for the benefit of the students.

The malignant style of questioning prevalent in medical schools features "techniques designed to humiliate the learner, such as 'guess what I'm thinking?' questions or testing knowledge so obscure that only the questioner would know the answer" (Kost & Chen, 2015, p. 20). Such malignant questioning, even when the questioning itself is not as painful, often brings about humiliation and shame because it is done in a very public setting. Students also can be hurt or ashamed if one student is singled out for a long period of time, or if a student's ideas are dismissed or ignored as the professor moves on to a new student to seek the desired answer (Kost & Chen, 2015).

In contrast, the Socrates of Plato's dialogues cares deeply about his interlocutors and is never looking for facts or one right answer. He does not engage in a fishing expedition of "guess what I'm thinking?" but focuses on the individual being questioned, trying to determine: What are this person's assumptions? What is he overlooking? Why did he give the answer or make the decision he just did? Indeed, Socrates often insists he does not know the answer to the questions at hand and wants to learn through dialogue with his interlocutor. Thus, true Socratic pedagogy is not merely about teaching and probing; it is also about a teacher and students learning together. The teacher is not expected or desired to have all the answers but to guide the questions and thinking to help all learn together.

Socratic Comportment

Today, we recognize that components essential to successful adult learning include "mutual respect; a safe and supportive educational environment; and challenging learners in a nonthreatening way" (Kost & Chen, 2015, p. 21). And 2,400 years ago, Socrates seemed to understand these same essential components for learning. Moreover, his calling and his greatest joy were teaching and learning with his students. He spent the majority of his time with Athens' youth. In Plato's dialogue *Charmides* (trans. 1992a), one of Socrates's first priorities when returning to Athens after a long absence is to inquire whether there are any promising youth ready to learn.

Certainly, Socrates was thought of as an annoying pest at times, especially by those in power whom Socrates encouraged the youth to question. But there is no doubt that Socrates's questioning came from a position of caring—for his students, for the city, for their citizenship in that city, a context not so different from nurse educators and their students today. Socrates's friends and students were devoted to him. At Socrates's execution, Phaedo and other friends gathered "all felt as if we had lost a father and would be orphaned for the rest of our lives" (Plato, 116a, trans. 1981e). It is clear that Socrates was a beloved teacher. His students as portrayed in Plato's dialogues note that he noted their reactions to a discussion and cared that they were learning and were not in too much distress (trans. 1981e).

When interlocutors do become frustrated, Socrates always emphasizes that he, too, is frustrated because he does not have the answers. He encourages his interlocutors to continue the dialogue so they can inquire together. Socrates believes he has a moral obligation to press his students to help them recognize their own mistaken beliefs or false assumptions. As he explains in Plato's *Theaetetus* (trans. 1990), "People have often before now got into such a state with me as to be literally ready to bite when I take some nonsense or other from them. They never believe that I am doing this in all good will; … I don't do this kind of thing out of malice, but because it is not permitted to me to accept a lie and put away truth" (151d).

Socrates as Stingray, Gadfly, and Midwife

Throughout Plato's works, he writes of different people making various analogies to describe Socrates and what it is like to have a conversation with him. Over 2,000 years later, these analogies can serve today's educators as models for how-to-be as teachers. Each of us can be a bit of the stingray, the gadfly, and the midwife.

Socrates' friend Meno, in the dialogue of the same name (Plato, trans. 1981d), finds himself in a frustrating conversation with Socrates about the nature of virtue and whether it can be taught like other subjects can. Meno offers an analogy to try to help Socrates understand how he feels when Socrates refuses to let Meno's answers be and continues pressing with more questions. He declares Socrates to be like a "torpedo fish," what we might call a stingray today. Meno seems to be partly joking, adding that Socrates even *looks* like a torpedo fish. But he is serious enough when he explains that like Socrates, the stingray "makes anyone who comes close and touches it feel numb" (80a–b). Socrates somewhat accepts this analogy, taking it in stride, but he argues it fits only in a limited way: "If the torpedo fish is itself numb and so makes others numb, then I resemble it, but not otherwise, for … I am more perplexed than anyone when I cause perplexity in others" (80c). Socrates is as likely to get "stung" himself as his students are, and Socrates believes that is just as it should be.

The most famous analogy for Socrates and his trademark questioning is the one devised by Socrates himself at his trial, as featured in Plato's *Apology* (trans. 1981a). He tells the gathered jurors that he was "attached to this city by the god … as upon a great and noble horse which was somewhat sluggish because of its size and needed to be stirred up by a kind of gadfly" (30e). Continuing with this analogy he adds, "I never cease to rouse each and every one of you, to persuade and reproach you all day long and everywhere I find myself in your company" (30e–31a). Socrates is here referring to the fact that he has used questioning every day to exhort his fellow Athenians to do good, to be good citizens. This unrelenting questioning, he believed, was his duty to Athens to keep it on a good path; his oft-irritating questioning was employed in service to others and to the greater good.

A nurse educator today has the same responsibility as Socrates to be a stingray and a gadfly, if not more so. In addition to Socrates' goal of helping his students grow into good citizens, nurse educators must also help students navigate a complex landscape of science, technology, ethics, and social interaction. A teacher who calls out a new nurse— respectfully, from a place of care—on a questionable decision, may sometimes seem like a stingray or a gadfly, but the teacher is nurturing that student and doing a service to the larger context of nursing practice and patient care.

Another analogy for Socrates is also one he offers up himself: He sees himself as a midwife. In Plato's *Theaetetus* (trans. 1990), Socrates explains that he is the son of a midwife, and while he does not help in pregnancy and delivery of children, he helps in the same sort of process in learning and the birthing of ideas. He explains that like the midwives of ancient Athens, he himself is barren, seeking to help those who are pregnant with ideas, such as students or others who are struggling with a concept or are on the verge of an important discovery. Socrates explains that he can help bring on delivery or relieve labor pains; he can help students know when they need to question or think through some of their ideas, and he can help them when they are lost or struggling. Also like midwives of his day, Socrates says he knows which couplings of ideas are likely to produce fertile offspring; he can help his students make connections between ideas and experiences to further their learning and understanding. Socrates says that his art is in one key way different from the traditional midwives' because he must also distinguish between "phantoms" and "realities," between errors and "fertile truth" once he has delivered another's ideas (149b–150c).

This image of Socrates as a midwife is extremely important because it allows us to see the other side of the stingray and the gadfly. Once he has stung (if necessary) a lazy horse or momentarily stunned a confused student, he continues to help that person through the painful process of moving from rejected assumptions or gaps in knowledge toward new ideas, connections, or pathways of thought. A nurse educator today is always a midwife as much as a gadfly. Out of caring for the students and patients, a teacher is obligated to press students with questions and poke around a bit for learning gaps. But just as importantly a teacher must help students think about what they already know and how it connects to their practice. The teacher can help them think through their own ideas and actions (correct or incorrect) to move them toward better knowledge, more confidence, and an increased ability to analyze their own ideas in the future.

Socrates as Teacher–Learner, Co-Inquirer

The consistent theme in all of these analogies for Socrates is that he does not know better than anyone else; he can get stung by his own stingray methods, and he can help others "deliver" ideas because he himself is barren, just like the midwives of his day. Consistently throughout Plato's dialogues, we see that Socrates is humble about his knowledge and wisdom. Plato tells his friend Theaetetus, "I am always asking questions of other people but never express my own views about anything, because there is no wisdom in me; and that is true enough … I am not in any sense a wise man; I cannot claim as the child of my own soul any discovery worth the name of wisdom" (150c, trans. 1990). And it is nearly always true that, as Socrates claims, he does not offer his own opinions on things. This holding back of his own ideas seems to be a key part of his pedagogy. In contemporary scholarship on teaching and learning, this holding back is sometimes referred to as a *Socratic veil*. Socrates does not want to give his students the answers—indeed he says he often does not have the answer—but instead wants to help them find the answers themselves.

Socrates' most elegant statement on his educational philosophy comes as a metaphor—Plato's famed Cave Allegory in the *Republic* (trans. 1992c). In the allegory, prisoners are shackled in a cave and have been there from birth. They see only shadows cast by a fire in the cave, and they believe these shadows to be reality. The journey out of the cave is difficult and painful, as the prisoners' eyes adjust to the light of the sun and they realize that now they are seeing truth, and everything they thought they knew before was misguided. In an incredibly poignant part of the story, Plato, writing this piece two decades after his beloved teacher's execution and choosing the words Socrates will say, has Socrates worry that if someone tries to go into the cave and bring the prisoners into the light, they may fight or even kill that person. Thus, Plato honors the sacrifice of his teacher who was only trying to help Athenians to learn to help themselves (514a–518b).

After Socrates finishes telling the story of the cave, he explains to his friends what the story tells us about education. Education is not a matter of putting knowledge into a soul ready to receive it. Rather, it is a matter of helping each person to realize he has knowledge within him, "that the power to learn is present in everyone's soul and that the instrument with which each learns is like an eye that cannot be turned around from darkness to light without turning the whole body" (518c). A teacher's job is to put students on the path leading out of the cave, and to catch them when they stumble, guide them when they cannot find their way, and comfort them when the journey becomes too difficult.

Socrates consistently emphasizes that he expects to learn as much from his students as they from him. At the end of the dialogue *Euthyphro* (Plato, trans. 1981c), he is disappointed that his dialogue partner on the subject of piety has suddenly remembered somewhere he has to be (a common escape plan for Socrates's interlocutors!) and says, "by going you have cast me down from a great hope I had, that I would learn from you the nature of the pious and the impious … and that I would be better for the rest of my life" (15e–16a). Similarly, in the *Theaetetus* (Plato, trans. 1990), Socrates tells his companions that the search for wisdom is a search inside each of themselves. He explains that when students discuss matters with him, they do not learn anything directly from him, but rather "they discover within themselves a multitude of beautiful things, which they bring forth into the light" (150d).

As educators today, we *can* learn from our students as we teach them. In nursing education, of course, the teacher has far more knowledge and experience on most subjects than the students are likely to have. And yet, students' inferior knowledge and skills do not prevent them from giving new insights on material being studied or on a situation with a patient. Sometimes students' novice outlook and lack of knowledge may free them to notice things an experienced instructor may have overlooked or forgotten. And like Socrates, nurse educators can hold back on giving answers or opinions, maintain a Socratic veil. Sometimes, of course, giving an answer will be the best thing for the student or patient. But more often, asking questions and letting the student find the answer him- or herself will be the better lesson. Socrates was a lifelong learner on a quest for knowledge and wisdom just as much as he was a teacher, and his best lesson to today's educators may well be that only through a constant desire to learn can one become a great teacher or a true lover of wisdom. And what a rewarding teaching experience it is to help students "discover within themselves a multitude of beautiful things, which they bring forth into the light" (Plato, 150d, trans. 1990).

SOCRATIC QUESTIONING

How and When to Start the Discussion

Socrates's trademark question-and-answer approach is often referred to as his *elenchus*, and it is important to understand that the elenchus is only part of the overall Socratic method we see modeled and described in Plato's works. Socratic questioning is certainly the most prominent aspect of the method, though, so we will start by examining this style of questioning before moving on to the rest of the method.

Socrates usually begins his questioning in response to some statement or action that makes Socrates wonder if the person has knowledge about a relevant issue. For instance, when he learns that the priest Euthyphro is about to prosecute his own father for murder (an act many Athenians would consider impious), Socrates wants to discuss piety with Euthyphro, to help Euthyphro determine what he does and does not know about piety and therefore pious actions. In a modern context, Socratic questioning often works well with a similar impetus. A teacher might say, "You did (or said) something that surprised me. Tell me your reasoning." Or, "You chose X instead of Y" or "You chose X when others might have been unsure what to do. Why did you do that?" By starting from a point of the student's statement or action, the student is already invested and engaged in the conversation, ready to explore and learn about the subject at hand.

Socrates's inquiries often move forward through a comparison of beliefs. He guides one person to compare his own various beliefs (Plato, *Euthyphro, Crito, Meno*) or guides a group to compare beliefs among themselves (Plato, *Phaedo, Republic*). Part of Socrates's goal in this comparison of beliefs is to look for inconsistencies or conflicting beliefs, because these often point the way to mistaken assumptions or gaps in knowledge. Socrates describes this comparison of beliefs to Theaetetus: "Our first aim will be to look at our thoughts themselves in relation to themselves, and see what they are—whether, in our opinion, they agree with one another or are entirely at variance" (Plato, 154e, trans. 1990). When Socrates finds conflicts between beliefs, he usually asks his interlocutors how they want to deal with the inconsistency. Do they want to abandon one of the things they have said in favor of another? Do they want to abandon an assumption Socrates has helped them realize they held?

In nursing, educators can check not only connectedness between beliefs but among all the other data and observations nurses must pay attention to. "Why did you do X?" "Because of Y." "But the patient also has a P situation. How does that connect? Is there a conflict there?" Students or new graduate nurses are often focused on tasks and specific skills and may not see the connections between bits of information. Engaging them in dialogues such as these examples can help students to be aware of what to notice when working with their patient and to make connections to see the whole picture of the patient's care needs.

Very consistently in Plato's works, Socrates insists that his dialogue partners must say what they truly believe. This is sometimes referred to as the "Say What You Believe" requirement (Vlastos, 1991, p. 113). Two typical statements of this requirement occur in the *Crito* and the

Charmides. Socrates asks Crito to "try to answer what I ask you in the way you think best" (Plato, 49a, trans. 1981b), and he asks Charmides, "I suppose you could express this impression of yours in just the way it strikes you?" (159a, trans. 1992a; see also *Euthyphro* 14e and *Laches* 193c). Even more pointedly, Socrates tells his friend Theaetetus: "if you answer 'Yes,' [just to avoid contradicting yourself] … the tongue will be safe from refutation but the mind will not" (154d, trans. 1990). This last quotation from Socrates lets us see the reason for the requirement. If students do not say what they actually believe, but instead say something to please the teacher or to avoid contradicting themselves, then the teacher is less able to help the student ferret out conflicts and inconsistencies in beliefs. In a classroom or clinical setting today, teachers should make clear to students that they want them to say what they really think or believe, not what they read in a book (but do not believe) or what they think the teacher wants to hear. The students must say what they believe because that is what needs to be tested. If a teacher thinks students are doing otherwise, the teacher should call them out on it!

Another consistent principle Socrates follows in his questioning is the Priority of Definition (Beversluis, 1987; Lesher, 1987; Nehamas, 1975). Socrates believes that he and his interlocutors have to start by looking for a definition of the thing in question before looking into aspects of that thing. When Meno wishes to know whether or not virtue is teachable (i.e., when he wants to know something *about* virtue), Socrates resists, saying, "I am so far from knowing whether virtue can be taught or not that I do not even have knowledge of what virtue itself is" (Plato, 71a, trans. 1981d). In the *Laches* (Plato, trans. 1992b), Socrates asks about courage, "If we are not absolutely certain what it is, how are we going to advise anyone as to the best method of obtaining it?" (190b–c). Socrates seems to believe that a definition or some other foundational point is necessary to anchor the conversation, to have not only a starting point but a point to return to later in the conversation. Definitions and foundational concepts also tend to be things that interlocutors can debate, shape, and explore together.

When teaching in today's classrooms and clinical settings, starting by asking for a definition may sometimes be appropriate. More likely, some other foundational principle will be a good starting point. "Shonda, what are the hematocrit levels we would expect to see with this patient?" Or "Lorie, in class you learned about the principles of NSAIDs (nonsteroidal anti-inflammatory drugs). Are there specific principles that you want to keep in mind when you give this medication to Mr. Rosen today?" Or, quite differently, "I see that you are frustrated and concerned, George. What would represent good care for you in this situation with this patient? Let's start from there." And then, after George responds, the teacher could follow up with more questions, helping George think through the priorities for providing good care for his patient. The teacher might then open up the question for the group of students: "What do you think represents good care in this situation?"

Using Analogies and Examples

Socrates often uses analogies to help his interlocutors clarify their thoughts. By putting questions into an easier, more recognizable context via an analogy, Socrates helps his co-inquirers more easily think through their own beliefs and assumptions. Not surprisingly, they find it far easier to think and talk about horse breeding or blacksmithing than to answer difficult questions about the nature of courage. By thinking about these analogous questions and situations, they are then more able to think carefully and directly about the question at hand.

Analogies can be used to pose a challenge as well. If an interlocutor seems too sure or comfortable of his statement or action, Socrates uses an analogy to get him to rethink his position. In the *Apology* (Plato, trans. 1981a), when Socrates's accuser at his trial, Meletus, boldly claims that all Athenians "make the young into fine good men" except for Socrates, Socrates demands, "Does this also apply to horses do you think? That all men improve them and one individual corrupts them? Or is quite the contrary true?" (25a–b).

Analogies can be very useful in clinical teaching, as they can help to make abstract concepts more concrete and help students understand what changes may be needed in specific situations. If a student is having trouble clarifying his or her thoughts on starting an IV, the instructor might ask, "Well, what if you were doing this with an elderly and frail patient? What if your patient is dehydrated? How would you adapt your IV insertion technique to meet the needs of this patient?" If the student does not understand what changes he or she should consider, the instructor might suggest, "Think of a sponge that has been sitting on the counter for a day and is all stiff. If you wanted to use it for cleaning, what would you do first?" Helping the student to think in concrete terms with an analogy such as the sponge may stimulate him or her to think of the potential for hydrating his or her patient to facilitate the IV start.

Likewise, if a student is having trouble seeing why his or her reasoning may be faulty or a decision in the simulation lab may be a problem, the instructor can introduce an analogy to help the student see the problem. Sometimes humorous analogies can be effective. For example, if a student is caring for a patient in the simulation lab who has a history of bed rest for several days and is complaining of abdominal pain with no obvious cause, the instructor may probe to see if the student considers the possibility of constipation. The instructor might ask: "What happens if you don't take the garbage out regularly?" (Beitz, 2013). The resulting humor is likely to help both the student and his or her peers remember to consider this possibility in the future. Thus, analogies can act as an anchoring concept, helping to create a type of "cognitive scaffolding" or framework upon which students can "hook" new information to previous understandings (Beitz, 2013).

Similar to his use of analogies, Socrates often gives examples to test his interlocutors' assumptions and reasoning. He gives examples that *should* fit what the interlocutor has said, but that do not *really* fit. For instance, if someone were to say to Socrates that "Love is an undying passion," Socrates might point to an obvious case in literature or life that most people would agree was love, but that perished or faded. In a nursing context, if a student says I did X because of Y, the teacher can ask, "Well, situation Z would also be Y—would you do that there?" For example, a student may say that it is important to get patients out of bed because it enhances blood circulation. The teacher might say: "Well, this patient has a suspected head injury. Would your rationale for getting patients out of bed hold for this patient?" If the answer to that question is "No," then the student would need to look for reasons for exceptions to the "get them out of bed" principle, such as identifying the need for bed rest in a patient with head injury to decrease further brain swelling.

Lack of Resolution: *Aporia* and Circling Back

Many of Socrates's conversations end without resolution. The Greek word for this lack of resolution is *aporia*—an impasse or puzzlement. Plato often dramatically brings attention to the situation of *aporia*: Socrates's companion suddenly has an appointment to keep or youths are run off by their guardians; in the *Symposium* (Plato, trans. 1989), the conversation is cut short by drunken revelers! *Aporia* is a key part of the Socratic process. Without a clear resolution, Socrates's dialogue partners are left to ponder the questions further on their own, or with each other, and may even feel driven to do so. In this way, the dialogue acts as a springboard for further dialogue and reflection.

Aporia will of course not be appropriate in conversations where a resolution is immediately necessary, such as urgent decisions for a patient's care. But in less pressing settings, nurse educators should resist the temptation to lead students to right answers or definite conclusions, because it is the thinking that is the goal; it is the journey that is valuable. The frustration or desire for further reflection and inquiry that result from *aporia* will show students the way to become lifelong learners and careful analysts of their situations going forward. Allowing a lack of resolution is an act of caring, like a parent running along holding onto the back of a young child's bike, then letting go so that the child can ride on his or her own. As Kost and Chen (2015) put it, "The ultimate aim of *elenchus* followed by *aporia* [is] to create a common ground—a state of curiosity—among everyone in the group. From there the group could begin a collective search for truth through further discussion" (p. 22).

The final Socratic questioning technique we should examine is his tendency to take the conversation in a circle or back to where it started. In the *Charmides* (Plato, trans. 1992a), Socrates insists, "Then start over again, Charmides" (160d); in the *Republic* (Plato, trans. 1992c), after many, many pages have gone by, Socrates suggests, "Let's return to the first things we said, since they are what led us here" (588b). This circling-back to the beginning or to an earlier point allows the current conversation to inform a previous one, and vice versa. And by moving with his dialogue partners back and forth, beginning from a similar point multiple times but following new paths, Socrates and his interlocutors are better able to catch their false assumptions and clarify their thoughts. This circling back technique is much like painting a wall, where with each stroke one overlaps the previous one while also covering new territory. And because the dialogue is a circle of sorts, it does not matter where one starts—in a complex clinical situation, many things are connected. Starting with one will lead to others, and then students can be invited to circle back to the beginning and re-examine their thoughts and tentative findings, making more connections as they go.

Socratic Dialogue in Today's Nurse Education Settings

Socrates's techniques—starting from where the student's thoughts and actions are, comparing beliefs, the "say what you believe" rule, priority of definition, analogies, examples, *aporia*, and circling back—are excellent strategies for clinical nurse educators to use in leading their students in Socratic discussion. It may also be helpful to look more closely at what such a discussion looks like in today's nursing setting. First and foremost, it is important for the teacher to explain the approach to students: Why questioning? What is the goal? Teachers should make very clear that the questions are directed toward the benefit of student learning and are intended in a respectful way. Teachers should further emphasize that during discussion, peers should show the same respect for the teacher and their peers.

It might be helpful to think of questions fitting into specific categories: exploratory, spontaneous, and focused (Tofade, Elsner, & Haines, 2013). Beginning with exploratory questions ("Can someone describe the situation to me?") puts students on a common ground and gives the teacher a good idea of what students know and understand. Spontaneous questions can then be asked to follow up on student responses. These questions cannot be planned ahead of time but should be drawn exclusively from the students' comments, challenging the students and asking them to clarify, think deeper, or consider implications. Then, if there is a topic of particular importance or interest, the teacher can ask more focused questions on that topic, inviting students to look at that part of the discussion in more detail.

Questions can be learner-centered or knowledge-centered (Kost & Chen, 2015). Knowledge-centered questions ("What did your physiology class tell you to expect with a patient like this?") can be interwoven occasionally into a discussion and can be a good way to test basic knowledge. The majority of questions, however, should be learner-centered, pressing students to reflect on their own beliefs, assumptions, and actions. Learner-centered questions can be "a series of progressively harder questions to encourage metacognition by helping a learner identify the contours of his or her knowledge base, including areas that need improvement" (Kost & Chen, 2015, p. 22).

In choosing questions, a teacher should aim for a good mix of comfortable questions (questions expected to fall within students' easy grasp) and harder questions. A Socratic discussion session should generally push students to a point *past* their comfort, confidence, and/or knowledge. Guiding them gently to that point of discomfort is what allows the students to discover gaps, recognize false assumptions, and question their own answers and decisions in a healthy, constructive way.

It may help the reader to look at some sample questions to illustrate these categories. "What were the relevant assessment findings?" would be a fairly comfortable, knowledge-centered, exploratory question. "What would you do based on these findings?" will prompt the student to move into slightly less comfortable territory. When the student responds, a question such as "Why was that your priority?" or "Why did you do X rather than Y?" will move the question into learner-centered, more difficult territory. This spontaneous question is a direct response to the answer the student gave. The student is now being asked to reflect on his or her own thinking and choices. If relevant or in line with learning goals, the teacher might then choose to focus on the student's response to this line of questions, inviting other students to provide their own thoughts on the matter.

In a Socratic discussion, exploratory questions can be planned ahead of time, but the majority of the teacher's questions must largely be determined by what the students say—a responsive, genuine inquiry in reaction to student actions and statements. And even starting or exploratory questions should not be overplanned; as Socrates often chose his discussion based on actions or decisions he witnessed, it is highly appropriate for a nurse educator to wait and choose the starting point of the discussion based on the happenings of the day in the classroom or simulation lab or on the hospital unit. The main goal is for the students to think, reflect, and learn. Going into a Socratic discussion session with too many specific content or skill goals in mind will hamper students' opportunities for genuine inquiry.

All of these techniques and guidelines are well and good for a teacher already comfortable leading discussions with a group of students. But many educators are used to imparting vast amounts of facts in order to cover all the content. These educators are most comfortable with lecture and other more planned teaching approaches. The transition to Socratic discussion can be a bit scary for these teachers. Researchers in a study that incorporated this approach with clinical instructors who were teaching new graduate nurses in a hospital setting found that after the instructors changed their teaching approach to Socratic discussion, they were initially quite uncomfortable, as they were used to providing answers, not having the students provide the answers (Sorrell, 2013). After several weeks of practice with the new approach, however, the instructors gradually became very enthusiastic about using it, as their students were actively engaged in learning. One clinical nurse educator who moved from a lecture approach to a teaching strategy of questioning with her students shared the following:

> It was stressed in this program [for new nurses] to use open-ended questions as a way of really being able to understand a nurse's thought process when it came to symptom identification and/or problem management. In the beginning, ... my first instinct was to either ask a simple yes/no question (one I felt they would get right to build confidence) or tell them the answer in the perceived setting of new material. I rarely do either now unless I feel the learner is really struggling.
>
> I feel that open-ended questions open the door to critical thinking. Open-ended questions force the ownership of the conversation back onto the learner. Instead of educators needing to ask the "right" question, the ownership is switched to the learner to embellish on the answer. It helps the learner think out loud and helps the educator identify learning gaps that can be closed.

Here are some tips that might help educators make the transition:

- Be comfortable with silence—do not answer your own questions! Do not change the question (unless it really just was not clear). Remember that students are *always* more uncomfortable with silence than you are.
- It can be good sometimes (not always) to let students think about a question before answering. Give them a chance to talk with each other or to do 5 minutes of writing on the question. For instance, they might write on: "What did we see in this video of the patient? What surprised or concerned you about what you saw?" Students could then share their responses, and those responses would serve as the starting point of discussion.

- If no student volunteers a response to a question, consider calling on a particular student; if that student cannot formulate a response, most likely another student will come to that student's rescue by speaking up. Ideally, "calling on someone in a non-threatening way tends to activate others who might otherwise remain silent" (Garlikov, n.d.).

- Do not overplan a class session. Have some idea of content or questions to be covered, but let the conversation flow where it wants to go; in this way, students are engaged and learning what they are ready and interested to learn.

With these tips in mind, and a bit of practice on Socrates's main techniques, a novice educator or an experienced lecturer can lead an engaging, productive discussion.

BEYOND TEACHER–STUDENT QUESTIONING: OTHER ASPECTS OF SOCRATIC PEDAGOGY

Teachers Telling Stories, Sharing Opinions

While Socrates's questioning is by far the most fundamental and famous part of his method, he also frequently makes use of stories to help his students think and learn. For instance, his friend Meno is troubled by the concern that learning of any sort might not be possible, because it is impossible to search for the things we do not know, for how will we know when we find them? As a teacher, Socrates is of course very invested in helping Meno find his way past this particular fear. To convince his friend that learning *is* possible, Socrates offers a myth, a story, one which he admits may not be accurate or true. He tells a story of how all souls learn all the knowledge before birth, then forget it when they are born; thus, learning is simply a matter of recollecting what has been forgotten. Even though Socrates admits the story may not be accurate or true, the spirit of it affects Meno and gives him a way of addressing his concerns. Meno responds, "Somehow, Socrates, I think that what you say is right" (Plato, 86a, trans. 1981d).

For nurse educators, stories of their own experiences, such as stories shared in this book, can lessen students' doubts, help them past a mental block, or help them make connections. Made-up stories—hypothetical situations, for instance—can serve almost like analogies, helping students think through a problem they are puzzling over. Stories have a power that fact-heavy lectures do not: They engage the imagination and creative thinking of the students. Thus, they can be ideal for helping students explore ethical questions or think through complex care scenarios.

While Socrates rarely shares his own views with his students and other dialogue partners, maintaining the position that he does not have the answers, on very special and important occasions he shares his beliefs and even tries to persuade others to agree with him. For example, Socrates has a firm belief in a "just deserts" version of an afterlife, and he tells the jurors at his trial that he knows his false accusers and impending execution cannot truly harm him: "Keep this one truth in mind, that a good man cannot be harmed either in life or in death, and that his affairs are not neglected by the gods" (Plato, 41d, trans. 1981a).

Quite similarly for nurse educators practicing Socratic pedagogy, it is important to withhold opinions and knowledge much of the time to give the students space to learn and inquire in their own way. But just as importantly, if a teacher holds a belief he or she thinks his or her students will be much better off believing themselves, then by all means he or she should share it. The teacher might, for instance, share and explain his or her belief that the patient always comes first, and what that means for him or her. Instructors should also take every opportunity to share their thoughts on their own teaching choices. For instance, if an instructor finds the need to step in on a procedure between a student nurse and a patient, the student will learn more (and be hurt less) if the instructor explains soon after, "Here's why I did that in there."

Peer Mentoring in Teams

Another supplement to teacher-guided Socratic questioning is peer-to-peer questioning. In a study by Duchscher (2001), teachers assigned one student in a clinical group to serve as the peer mentor for the day. Peer mentors were then "encouraged to use critical thinking skills, reflective questioning, and mutual collaboration in their interaction with students" (p. 60). Duchscher reports that students found this peer mentoring arrangement to be "mutually supportive, cooperative, and collaborative" (p. 60). The peer mentors themselves appreciated "the value placed on their knowledge and experience, claiming to have grown in both the diligence and precision with which they approached their own practice, and in the personal confidence with which they made clinical and practice decisions…. They identified a profound sense of professional responsibility that they claimed was unmatched in other clinical learning experiences" (p. 60).

Effectively, in this study, one student at a time was invited to play the Socratic role, to mentor and guide peers through questioning and critical reflection. Peer-to-peer questioning has a special value: "By learning how to ask questions of other students and of themselves," students learn not "merely to follow someone else's lead, but to lead others and to lead themselves in critical analysis" (Bloch-Schulman, 2012, p. 22). This kind of learning is exactly what is sought in the Carnegie study—going beyond answering questions to thinking about *what questions to ask* will make students better able to reason in changing clinical situations, to engage in critical, creative, and scientific reasoning (Benner et al., 2010).

Opportunities for Reflection and Meta-Cognition

Socrates consistently encourages his friends and students to continue a given discussion among themselves. After a short teaching session with a young boy, Socrates says to Meno, "These opinions have now just been stirred up in him like a dream, but if he were repeatedly asked these same questions in various ways, you know that in the end his knowledge about these things would be as accurate as anyone's" (Plato, 85c–d, trans. 1981d). Nursing students encouraged to revisit and reflect on previous inquiries will be working to "tie down" their beliefs and classroom content, transforming these beliefs and content into more confident and reliable knowledge by continuing to ferret out faulty assumptions and knowledge gaps and revealing connections between concepts and ideas.

When students are left in a state of *aporia* and then encouraged (or required) to circle back and re-examine the inquiry, they are being shown how to develop lifelong habits of re-examination and reflection. This circling back can take many forms. The teacher may guide the students in a reflection on the discussion from the previous day in which students question each other about what was said. A teacher might ask students to write a short reflective piece immediately after a class discussion or clinical conference. Or students might be assigned partners, and their homework could be to interview each other—each one taking a turn at playing Socrates—on their thoughts about that day's lesson and discussion. The students would then each write up a reflection on those two interviews, giving them a chance for meta-cognition on the subject at hand, a chance to reflect on their own and their partner's thoughts. Students who have done such an exercise with paired interviews and meta-cognition report deeper understanding, more connections with material learned, and better retention (Dinkins, 2014).

CONCLUSION

Trying a new—and perhaps radically different—style of teaching can be frightening, no doubt. And many students may report that they prefer to learn in a more passive way ("Just tell me what to do so I can be sure to do it right"). But for the type of teaching that clinical nurse educators are responsible for, it is critical to give students many opportunities for active learning to help them develop clinical reasoning and multiple ways of thinking. As a novice nurse educator, you are in an excellent position to try a new way of helping students to think like a nurse because you are not wedded to the traditional approach of imparting facts to students. Most likely, even a first attempt at Socratic questioning will find students engaged and excited to be treated as co-inquirers into questions of best practices. And the students most resistant to analyzing and questioning their own beliefs and actions on the floor or in the simulation lab are probably those who need it most. What better service to those students than to be a gadfly-midwife and stir them out of their overconfidence, confusion, or lack of self-reflection?

Socratic pedagogy is so incredibly flexible, able to adapt to the setting and subject, that it is an ideal way to teach skills; knowledge; clinical reasoning; and critical, creative, and ethical thinking. Through Plato's writings, Socrates gives us a shining example of what a teacher can and should be. He guides the people of Athens to question their own beliefs and assumptions so that they can make better decisions about how to be good citizens. He is also just as open to learning from his students as he is to teaching them. If today's nurse educators strive for similar interactions with their students, they may become not only better teachers but better learners as well.

Questions for Reflection

1. What worries you about switching to a more Socratic approach in your clinical teaching? Can you find a colleague or teaching partner with whom you can talk through your concerns?
2. Thinking back on previous teaching experiences (where you were the teacher or the student), describe a time when a Socratic approach would have been welcome or helpful and articulate why it would have been.
3. Imagine a scenario in which your student is overlooking a key part of the patient's presenting symptoms. What kind of questions can you ask the student (individually or in a group) to help him or her recognize what's being overlooked?
4. Your group of students just finished a rotation in the rehabilitation unit. They practiced a lot of new skills and hopefully solidified some relevant knowledge. What is a writing prompt you could give to help them reflect on their experience and their learning?
5. Your students tell you they would be more comfortable if you would prioritize giving them information instead of asking them questions. They are nervous about getting the answers right. What can you say to reassure them? How do you explain to them your rationale for teaching through questions?

REFERENCES

Beitz, J. M. (2013). Power up your patient education with analogies and metaphors. *Wound Care Advisor*. Retrieved from woundcareadvisor.com/power-up-your-patient-education-with-analogies-and-metaphors_vol2-no5/

Benner, P., Hughes, R. G., & Sutphen, M. (2008). Clinical reasoning, decision making, and action: Thinking critically and clinically (Chapter 6). In R. G. Hughes (Ed.), *Patient safety and quality: An evidence-based handbook for nurses*. Rockville, MD: Agency for Health Care Research and Quality. Retrieved from www.ncbi.nlm.nih.gov/books/NBK2643/

Benner, P., Sutphen, M., Leonard, V., & Day, L. (2010). *Educating nurses: A call for radical transformation*. San Francisco, CA: Jossey-Bass.

Beversluis, J. (1987). Does Socrates commit the Socratic fallacy? *American Philosophical Quarterly*, 24(3), 211–223.

Bloch-Schulman, S. (2012). The Socratic method: Teaching and writing about philosophy's signature pedagogy. In N. L. Chick, A. Haynie, R. A. R. Gurung, & A. R. Regan (Eds.), *Exploring more signature pedagogies: Approaches to teaching disciplinary habits of mind* (pp. 15–26). Sterling, VA: Stylus.

Boghossian, P. (2003). How Socratic pedagogy works. *Informal Logic, 23*(2), 17–25.

Dinkins, C. S. (2014). *Socratic shared inquiry as a model for assessing student learning outcomes.* Unpublished study.

Duchscher, J. E. B. (2001). Peer learning: A clinical teaching strategy to promote active learning. *Nurse Educator, 26*(2), 59, 60.

Garlikov, R. (n.d.). The Socratic method: Teaching by asking instead of by telling. Retrieved from www.garlikov.com/Soc_Meth.html

Kost, A., & Chen, F. M. (2015). Socrates was not a pimp: Changing the paradigm of questioning in medical education. *Academic Medicine, 90*(1), 20–24.

Lesher, J. H. (1987). Socrates' disavowal of knowledge. *Journal of the History of Philosophy, 25,* 275–288.

Marlow, E., Nosek, M., Lee, Y., Young, E., Bautista, A., & Hansen, F. T. (2015). Nurses, formerly incarcerated adults, and Gadamer: Phronesis and the Socratic dialectic. *Nursing Philosophy, 16*(1), 19–28.

Nehamas, A. (1975). Confusing universals and particulars in Plato's early dialogues. *Review of Metaphysics, 29,* 287–306.

Plato. (trans. 1981a). *Apology. Five dialogues* (G. M. A. Grube, Trans.). Indianapolis, IN: Hackett.

Plato. (trans. 1981b). *Crito. Five dialogues* (G. M. A. Grube, Trans.). Indianapolis, IN: Hackett.

Plato. (trans. 1981c). *Euthyphro. Five dialogues* (G. M. A. Grube, Trans.). Indianapolis, IN: Hackett.

Plato. (trans. 1981d). *Meno. Five dialogues* (G. M. A. Grube, Trans.). Indianapolis, IN: Hackett.

Plato. (trans. 1981e). *Phaedo. Five dialogues* (G. M. A. Grube, Trans.). Indianapolis, IN: Hackett.

Plato. (trans. 1989). *Symposium* (A. Nehamas & P. Woodruff, Trans.). Indianapolis, IN: Hackett.

Plato. (trans. 1990). *Theaetetus* (M. J. Levett & M. Burnyeat, Trans.). Indianapolis, IN: Hackett.

Plato. (trans. 1992a). *Charmides. Laches and Charmides* (R. K. Sprague, Trans.). Indianapolis, IN: Hackett.

Plato. (trans. 1992b). *Laches. Laches and Charmides* (R. K. Sprague, Trans.). Indianapolis, IN: Hackett.

Plato. (trans. 1992c). *Republic* (G. M. A. Grube & C. D. C. Reeve, Trans.). Indianapolis, IN: Hackett.

Rogge, M. M. (2001). Transforming pathophysiology instruction through narrative pedagogy and Socratic questioning. *Nurse Educator, 26*(2), 66–69.

Sorrell, J. M. (2013). Evaluating the use of human patient simulation (HPS) to improve critical thinking competencies and perceived self-confidence of new graduate nurses in the intensive care unit. Unpublished study.

Tedesco-Schneck, M. (2013). Active learning as a path to critical thinking: Are competencies a roadblock? *Nurse Education in Practice, 13*, 58–60.

Tofade, T., Elsner, J., & Haines, S.T. (2013). Best practice strategies for effective use of questions as a teaching tool. *American Journal of Pharmaceutical Education. 77*(7), Article 155. Retrieved from www.ncbi.nlm.nih.gov/pmc/articles/PMC3776909/

Vlastos, G. (1991). *Socrates, ironist and moral philosopher*. Ithaca, NY: Cornell University Press.

PART III

Learning From First-Hand Narratives

CHAPTER 7

Reflections of a Clinical Educator in a Baccalaureate Nursing Program

Lorena Jung

Education is not the filling of a pail but the lighting of a fire.
—William Butler Yeats

I earned a bachelor's of science in nursing from the University of Virginia and obtained my first job working as a night shift hospice care nurse at a local community hospital. This felt like a good match for my first job because I was not seeking a fast-paced environment to start out in as a novice nurse. In this first job I appreciated the opportunity to strengthen clinical skills over time as well as observe the deeply caring, compassionate, and holistic approach to the care of terminally ill patients. Effective communication, teamwork, and patient/family collaboration were also well practiced on this unit. All of these skills are taught during school but to have actually witnessed them in the workplace was a good learning experience for a new nurse.

I later worked at the bedside on units such as oncology and medical–surgical nursing. I eventually earned a master's degree and then worked in a community health/quality improvement position at an international health clinic in Seattle, Washington. Working with vulnerable, international patient populations continues to be a passion of mine. Later, when I was working on an oncology research unit at the National Institutes of Health (NIH) patient care center, I was invited to become a nurse educator. I was attending school part time to earn my nursing doctoral degree and had reduced my workload at NIH. The school of nursing (SON) contacted me midsemester and asked if I might be available to take over a community health clinical group that had been "abandoned" by one of their clinical instructors. After the first few weeks into the semester, the instructor simply vanished, never to be heard from by her students or the SON again. The clinical coordinator was seeking a replacement and had reached out to several graduate students with community health experience. Despite a full schedule, the new role sparked my interest and I agreed to take on my first clinical instructor position.

DECISION TO BECOME A NURSE EDUCATOR

One of the primary reasons for me to become a nurse educator was to share nursing knowledge with new nurses. I also wanted to guide students toward success. I remember being an average student throughout my whole life and never dreamed that someday I would be holding a nursing doctoral degree. I remember specific incidents from elementary school through college where teachers spoke negative or positive words that left lifelong impressions.

Upon entering graduate school, I suddenly decided I did not want to continue on as a mediocre student and instead, I wanted to put forth my best efforts academically. I worked diligently on the first nursing course paper that was due. The day our papers were returned, I remember the professor saying, "Lorena, I was surprised, you write well!" She will probably never know that I too was surprised. I felt like a hidden talent had been revealed; I felt motivated to keep improving my writing skills. This professor's words stuck with me throughout my graduate studies. If she had not mentioned anything on that day, I would probably have never developed a love for writing or a desire to write a lengthy dissertation.

Words can either bring harm or encouragement at any stage of education. I knew I would really like to teach in a nursing program when I realized how simple encouragement could motivate a student. Words do not cost anything, and they make an immense impact on a student's future. Now, as an educator, I find there seems to be at least one or two students each semester who just need to hear positive affirmation to help keep them going. I hope that my words can influence them in the same way my own professor's words strengthened me years ago.

One of the major benefits that I look forward to as a nurse educator is the sharing of knowledge and exchange of creative ideas. I do not have an authoritarian style of teaching. I believe that I have just as much to learn from students as they do from me. Some of my students have more experience than I do; I welcome their sharing of experiences since we all learn from them. Many meaningful teaching or learning experiences have occurred through this collaborative approach.

One major concern that may arise with a belief in a collaborative student/teacher learning approach is the possibility of students crossing boundaries and hijacking teaching authority. Students may misinterpret the collaborative learning style and perceive the teacher as being too kind and easily manipulated. However, through the years, I have adapted to each group of students and their learning needs. I have had to learn to become more assertive when a student has crossed certain boundaries, such as demonstrating unprofessional behaviors. Students who lash out are often very stressed or overwhelmed. I have come to realize that I am not meant to be the target because when I respond in a firm, professional manner, the student typically cools off and apologizes. Trust and respect can be gained over time and when a particularly challenging student wants to stay in touch with me after the semester is over, that is one of the sweetest rewards of being a nurse educator.

STARTING AS A NURSE EDUCATOR

My very first day as a nurse educator started in the community health clinical rotation. I was assigned to a group of students midsemester who were placed in school health settings throughout a large-sized county. Their "home base" was located at the county's health department. It was here that I first met these students when we convened for post-clinical discussion. Even though I had earned my master's in science of nursing degree in community health, I wondered if I possessed enough knowledge to share with the students. I was also worried that a question might be asked that I might not be able to answer, even though today I know it is all right to not have all the answers. I also hoped that students would like, respect, and accept me.

I was pleasantly surprised during this first post conference that the students were smiling and happy to see me. Apparently their previous clinical instructor did not show up for postclinical discussion for several weeks in a row. Even though the students dutifully appeared every week to share experiences and learn about each other's clinical day, they would be left waiting and wondering what to do next. After I introduced myself, the students each shared their clinical experiences and we went over clinical expectations. Another pleasant surprise was when students shared how they looked forward to submitting assignments to me since they had not received feedback from their earlier submissions. At the end of the semester, I felt fortunate to have had a fairly smooth first-time teaching experience and I looked forward to the semesters ahead.

One of my first positive experiences as a nurse educator occurred during an intense, 5-week summer medical–surgical clinical rotation. The students and I worked closely together Monday through Thursday from 7:30 to 4:00 p.m.. In this group, there was a young man who had a major attitude that he forgot to leave at home. During orientation, Mark interrupted me and started other conversations while I was still talking. Afterward, I approached Mark and asked him if he was upset about anything specific and offered him the opportunity to switch clinical placements if he did not want to work with me. I made it clear we would be working closely together in the weeks to come. I did not want any communication barriers during an intense clinical experience. Mark responded gruffly that he might consider switching sites and that he felt the rift forming between us was "a cultural thing," the "cultural thing" being based on my Asian background versus his White American background. Surprisingly, he was not aware that I was born and raised in the United States, English is my primary language, and I crave chicken soup when I get sick.

Eventually, Mark decided he would not switch clinical groups and gradually understood I was a supportive instructor. He was smart and a meticulous caregiver. One of his classmates reported to me that Mark had found a small pressure ulcer on an elderly patient's back during a bed bath. This patient had been hospitalized for more than a few days and was given previous baths but no one else had found the beginning sore. I was proud of Mark's growing clinical skills and despite our rough beginning and his initial hesitancy, I praised him for taking care of his patients skillfully. In turn, he seemed to receive my words of encouragement with an open mind and I began to witness an angry heart soften.

Mark shared stories of his tough childhood and ongoing challenges outside of school. I believe he was motivated to become a nurse because he truly cared for people. At the end of the summer rotation, I offered to serve as a reference for each of my students during job searches. On our last clinical day, my students and I went out for a celebration lunch. Mark brought me a bouquet of flowers and sweets. It made the past 5 grueling clinical weeks all worth it. I was touched when a few months later Mark asked me to be a reference for him. We addressed personal differences and today I am proud to call him a colleague and friend.

The greatest challenge in deciding whether or not nursing education was the right career option for me has occurred during periods of personal financial instability. Unfortunately, in nursing, pay does not always reflect one's experience and the extensive time required to perform effectively. A master's or doctoral-level prepared nurse may end up earning less in academia compared to a bachelor's prepared nurse working at a large health system. Many of my students who graduate and begin their careers may start earning entry-level salaries that are higher than mine.

Despite those periods of financial struggle and the temptation to possibly earn more by switching over to a clinical setting, I do not regret the path that I have chosen. I believe I have a purpose as a nurse educator and it is a career path that is personally and professionally fulfilling.

RESOURCES NEEDED

It took me at least three semesters to get adjusted and feel comfortable in the clinical nurse educator role. A strong faculty support system and available university resources for struggling students, such as academic tutoring, made the difference for me. Now, as a full-time nurse educator, I reflect on what was most helpful to me in transitioning to this new role.

Faculty support and mentorship were crucial. I have taught clinical courses at various nursing programs in the surrounding area. Some SONs offered a formal mentorship matching program while other programs were more informal and a mentor was not necessarily matched to a new faculty member. If a mentor was not assigned, I would seek to find my own. It was also helpful to have an in-service regarding university services and supplemental learning resources available to students. I would often seek the assistance of the clinical or course coordinator for clinical-related questions. If a student was struggling academically, I would work with both the clinical coordinator and the student's advisor.

Clinical evaluation tools and grading rubrics were invaluable. Students could visualize progress and grasp a clear understanding of areas in need of improvement. Holding a monthly brown bag luncheon for new faculty and mentors or establishing a website link with teaching resources and a Q&A discussion board may also be helpful. One of the most important qualities that a nursing program can offer is strong support for new educators. This begins with strong leadership that is collaborative with both faculty and students.

CLINICAL NURSE EDUCATOR ROLE

When teaching clinical, I prepared by reading the course chapters that corresponded to the students' syllabus plan. I also ran literature searches on databases to search for new research-based publications that might serve as supplemental learning material. During postclinical discussions, if a student brought up a question that did not necessarily align with the course content but was still relevant to nursing practice, then we searched the literature together to find updated, evidence-based articles that supported the clinical practices observed. When teaching clinical, I am concerned primarily with providing enough supervision and guidance to ensure students are practicing patient care safely. At the end of the day, hoped-for outcomes include well-cared-for patients and students who have learned at least one new skill.

I make patient assignments based on how well the student demonstrates clinical skills, knowledge level, organization, and time management. If a student progresses over the course of the semester and wants the challenge of caring for multiple patients, which mirrors a true workplace experience, then I assign up to three patients during the one clinical shift. Those students who are ready for this more realistic assignment are usually well prepared and end up performing effectively.

I believe in incorporating updated, evidence-based knowledge and practice into my teaching. There is often a disconnect between research evidence and actual nursing practice. An important role of the nurse educator is to bridge this disconnect, translating science into actual practice. Each semester, I hope to instill in my students a greater appreciation for nursing research. Some students have expressed a burgeoning interest in returning to a focus on research after gaining clinical experience.

When a student feels encouraged and realizes his or her own strengths and potential to be a successful nurse, then I know I have accomplished my goal of making a difference in that student's life. I do not seek to be recognized by my students in a formal manner; my only hope is that I may have spoken a few words at a timely moment in their lives that might impact them as they advance in their careers. At the end of each semester, I encourage students to consider returning to school for graduate studies, as learning is a lifelong process and does not stop after graduation, especially in health care.

LESSONS LEARNED FROM TRANSITIONING TO THE CLINICAL NURSE EDUCATOR ROLE

I feel that my graduate (MSN and PhD) degrees helped to prepare me for the nurse educator role. Graduate studies provided additional knowledge as well as enhanced critical thinking skills, which were foundational in leading, teaching, and guiding students throughout their course semester. If I could rewind a few years back, I would seriously consider obtaining a teaching certificate for additional preparation. I would be interested in studying more in-depth student learning styles and innovative teaching strategies.

Multiple factors have influenced my decision to remain in a nurse educator role. Strong family support is crucial, as my husband encourages me to establish my nursing career in an area that I enjoy. Although years of education are not reflected in my annual salary, I appreciate that my husband is accepting and understands that I feel called to teach. Another driving factor has been the ongoing desire to inspire and encourage students to reach their goals. I always look forward to adding another group of bright, caring nurses to our profession. Nurse educators are in a prime position to prepare future quality caregivers.

CHAPTER 8

Reflections of a Clinical Educator in an Associate Degree Nursing Program

Felicia Michelle Glasgow

The function of education is to teach one to think intensively and to think critically. Intelligence plus character—that is the goal of true education.

—Dr. Martin Luther King, Jr.

These influential words guide not only my thoughts and behaviors as a nurse in general, but also my instructional practices as a nurse educator. This quote has been a beacon of light illuminating my own educational path for the past 23 years. As an expert clinician, this quote became a standard rule by which I measured my knowledge base, professional conduct, and manner in which I delivered care to patients and families. Over the years, this inspiring quote became an instrument in my character development toolkit and has helped me evolve into the nursing professional—specifically, the nurse educator—I am today. For me, becoming a nurse educator was about not only teaching my students how to think at a comprehensive level, but also teaching them how to practice by principles that would allow them to construct a robust foundation upon which they could build their own professional character.

At the age of four, not knowing why I said it, or even where the thought came from, I remember looking up at my mother and saying, "I am going to be a nurse when I grow up. I want to help people help themselves." With a warm spirit and encouraging smile, my mother looked down into my wide brown eyes and said, "Baby, you can be whoever you want to be." That very moment was the first of many educational lessons to come. Today, over four decades later, I stand in my truth of becoming a nurse; one who helps other people to help themselves.

After completing a short period in the United States military, I decided to fulfill my dream of becoming a nurse. I entered the nursing profession as a licensed vocational nurse (LVN) and worked in long-term health care for 4 years. I provided direct hands-on task-oriented care to the geriatric patient population and their family members, and occasionally functioned in the role of a unit charge nurse for unlicensed health care staff. I took great pride in my role as a LVN and served my patients, their families, and my staff with a sense of humility.

Though being a LVN who took care of others gave me a sense of self-effacement, it did not quench my eagerness to strive for a more integral role in the nursing profession. I wanted to do more in nursing. I knew within myself that there was more to me—that there were more knowledge and skills for me to learn, and work for me to do at an advanced level. So, in search of personal gratification and professional growth, I made the decision to leave the long-term care setting to seek employment in an acute care setting. I quickly learned that opportunities were limited in acute care for nurses in the LVN role. I applied for several nursing positions in various acute care facilities only to be met with two very common answers, "We are not hiring LVNs at this time, maybe check back at a later date" or "We are looking to hire RNs at this time."

Frustrated, and unwilling to take no for an answer, I returned to college and earned an associate of applied science nursing degree. I was hired for a medical–surgical unit and mother–baby postpartum unit at one of the same hospitals that had earlier rejected me. I soon recognized that as a RN, my nursing experiences changed from performing simple bedside tasks and being an occasional shift leader to more comprehensive responsibilities. As I began to witness the level of influence my professional nurse teaching had on positive changes occurring in the lives of my patients, their families, and my professional work environment, I knew I wanted to be an educator.

I could see that my approach to sharing health information with others empowered them to improve their own circumstances. Patients were changing their lifestyle behaviors, which contributed to quicker wound healing, decreased hypertension numbers, and blood sugar levels declining to acceptable ranges. I witnessed new parents display more confidence and less fear when taking their newborns home. My nursing peers and other colleagues shared how my unit in-services helped to increase their professional knowledge base and improve their clinical practice skills. These were defining events that helped to inspire me to further my education and become a full-time nurse educator.

I wanted to become a trailblazer in nursing, empowering others through knowledge and experiences so that they could develop wisdom and understanding about their health and make life-altering changes to their health status. So back to school! Four years after earning my associate degree in nursing, I earned a bachelor of science in nursing (BSN) degree and transitioned from working in the acute hospital care setting to working as a community-based nurse educator for a local university area health education center (AHEC). In this role, I was able to help facilitate professional nursing educational programs, multidisciplinary health care seminars, and preventive community health fairs. For 5 years, I traveled through seven underserved counties empowering individuals who had little to no health knowledge, health insurance, or immediate access to health care services. Once again, I witnessed how education helped people make decisions that led to life-altering changes in their circumstances. The experience fueled my motivation to learn more and to teach more. Two years after earning my BSN, I returned to the same university and earned a master of nursing science (MNSc) degree.

NURSE EDUCATOR AS PRECEPTOR

After completing my master's degree, I continued to work as a community-based nurse educator and also as a nurse preceptor for nursing students who were seeking to earn their BSN from the same university in which I had earned my degrees. As a nurse preceptor, I was able to employ my years of diverse nursing clinical experiences, knowledge, and practice skills and to guide students through both simple and complex learning opportunities. Though the experience was enjoyable, I quickly realized that precepting students was not easy.

During each of my preceptor rotations I generally worked with two or three students at the same time. I learned that students in the clinical setting brought with them their own learning styles, educational beliefs and values, communication methods, and one common barrier to learning how to interact with patients: fear. Though most of my students were excited about their first clinical rotation, they were hesitant to engage with patients. As an experienced nurse working with other experienced nurses, I had not been aware of the level of fear that students brought with them to the clinical setting. I did not think about their fears or individual needs, but just what I needed to teach them about implementing safe and competent nursing skills.

This all changed 3 days into my role as a preceptor when one of my students, whom I will refer to as Lauren, asked a very simple, yet matter-of-fact question. Standing in front of me with her hands extended forward and shaking, Lauren asked, "Have you noticed my shaking hands today?" Somewhat caught off guard by her question, I stood staring at Lauren, trying to process her question. So many thoughts were running through my mind. I had no idea why she had asked me such a question. I responded honestly, saying "I am sorry, no I had not noticed." Lauren then explained that over the course of the past 3 clinical days she had experienced a level of fear when caring for her patients, despite knowing she was doing so under my supervision. She also explained that because of the way she was feeling, she did not think she was performing at her best.

As an experienced nurse in a preceptor role, I felt terrible that I had not detected Lauren's level of fear. I started to question my ability to be an effective clinical preceptor and whether or not my lack of experience in working with students had contributed to her fear. This incident was an indicator to me that I needed to pause and have a very open discussion with all of my students about how they were feeling in the clinical environment. I also needed to learn about how they thought I was performing as their preceptor. Each student was able to provide me with valuable insight into how they were feeling. Each student stated that they felt their fear negatively influenced their performances. They also shared that they knew I was super focused on providing them great clinical experiences, but I did not seem to be aware of the "I am afraid or anxious" cues they were displaying. I learned a crucial lesson—that awareness is an essential component to effectively teaching others.

As an experienced clinician, I had forgotten about how intimidating a patient care environment could be for the first time. But as a new preceptor myself, responsible for the learning experiences and outcomes of students, I could certainly understand my students' position because this unfamiliar territory also caused me some degree of fear. I found out in 3 short clinical days that I had just as much to learn from my students as they had to learn from me, and that awareness can bring about positive changes in students' clinical experiences. From that point forward, I used this lesson to shape my teaching approach. At the start of each new rotation I would ask students to describe their feelings about the clinical environment and whether they were experiencing some level of fear. I am very grateful that on that third day of clinical Lauren challenged me to become a better educator.

My role as a preceptor surpassed my wildest dream. I loved it! I loved witnessing each time one of my preceptees experienced an "a-ha" learning moment, or when one would come running from a patient's bedside exclaiming, "I did it! I can't believe I did it!" The enthusiasm my students exhibited as they grew into their own professional identity fed my desire to teach. My sense of purpose to become a nurse educator became clearer to me with each student I precepted. I knew without a doubt my purpose in the field of nursing was to help shape the minds and professional behaviors of the next generation of nurses through the power of education. I knew I could help teach students entering the nursing profession, or those advancing in the nursing profession, to think intensively and critically, and to develop the professional character needed to help change lives. Knowing that I had finally identified that integral part of the nursing profession that I had yearned for so many years was a priceless feeling.

NURSE EDUCATOR IN A SCHOOL OF NURSING

Excited and afraid at the same time, I decided I wanted to teach students in a structured nursing program, who in return would go forth and teach on a global level. In my mind, this would be my greatest contribution to the nursing profession. Therefore, I applied for a full-time faculty position at a local community college. I started out as both a classroom and clinical educator. Though being full of enthusiasm and eager to step into my new role, I began to experience some anxiety, fear, and doubt. I was concerned that despite my years of professional nursing education and direct experiences with students as a nurse preceptor, I would not be able to live up to the expectations of my nursing leaders, but more importantly, my students.

The night prior to my first day of teaching, I paced the floor, worrying. At times, I would think that taking on this new role was a big mistake and that I was better at teaching patients and staff in the clinical arena. I would then counteract those thoughts by thinking how would I know whether I was good at instructing students in a nursing program if I never tried? Other worries crept in: "What if I pronounce my words incorrectly?" "What if students ask me questions I can't answer?" "As an African American woman, am I culturally diverse enough to teach a multicultural body of students?" "How will students perceive my teaching methods?"

All of these questions intensified my stress level. However, I was able to reflect, and draw a level of confidence from my teaching experiences leading up to this position. By changing the way I was thinking, I was able to change the way I was feeling. I was ready to jump into my new nurse educator (faculty) role.

As a new full-time nurse educator, I quickly learned that nurse educators wore multiple hats and performed many duties throughout the course of a day. In addition to lecture in the classroom, teaching basic foundational nursing skills in the lab, and facilitating students' hands-on and observational clinical experiences in hospitals, clinics, and long-term care facilities, I assisted with administrative duties, such as program evaluations, committee participation, faculty advisement, and curriculum revisions.

In my initial role as a classroom educator, I taught several first-level courses, including basic nursing concepts, health assessment, basic nursing skills, and nursing foundations. Each course enrolled approximately 40 to 50 new students per semester. These courses had a concurrent simulation nursing skills lab component in which I worked 2 to 3 days out of the week with other faculty to teach students skills, such as physical assessment, medication administration, dressing changes, sterile techniques, and patient charting. Once students demonstrated mastery of the skills, they moved into real-life clinical settings, where they performed nursing tasks under the direct supervision of nursing faculty, learning to translate nursing theory into clinical practice as they worked with patients. The average student to faculty ratio in the clinical rotation was 10:1.

Classroom Teaching

On my first day as a classroom educator, I arrived at the nursing building and literally leaped out of my car in anticipation of starting my day and my new career path. As I entered the halls of the nursing department, I noticed faculty, staff, and some students scurrying around trying to prepare for an expected busy day. I was greeted with smiles and welcomes from colleagues, and nervous stares and fidgety hands from students. I thought about how I was feeling just the night before, and quickly concluded that the students were just as anxious and afraid of the unknown as I was.

I made my way to my office and after an hour of organizing my office space, I entered the classroom to meet the new cohort of nursing students I would be teaching for the semester. Once again, those previous intruding questions began to enter my mind. As I anxiously entered the classroom, students were engaged in multiple sidebar conversations. I quickly gained control of the learning environment, introduced myself, called the roll, and began to present the course information and class expectations. After all the beginning course formalities were completed, I proceeded with my first official lecture. My voice quivered, my knees shook, and I could literally feel beads of sweat trail down my spine. I thought to myself, "Am I going to make it through this?" Not knowing if I would, I paused in the middle of my lecture and asked my students "Is there anyone else in the classroom as nervous as I am?" In unison, students' hands went up all over the classroom, and in that very moment, I found strength in realizing I was not alone. I smiled at my students, realigned my thoughts, and completed my lecture.

After class was over, I stayed to answer questions for those students who lingered. I remember one student in particular; I'll call her Sun, because she was the brightest part of my first day. She was the last student to leave the class. Slowly, and appearing unsure of herself, she approached me and shared how much she enjoyed my lecture and teaching methods and the reasons she wanted to become a nurse. In all that she shared, her most profound statement was: "I want to learn everything I can about nursing so I can take care of people the right way, and help them to help themselves." I suddenly remembered when I was 4 years old and made the same declaration to my mother. I then looked Sun in her eyes, and with the same warm smile and encouraging spirit my mother had validated my dream so many years before, I told Sun, "You can be whoever you want to be." In that moment, I recognized that

I had been presented with a precious opportunity and a gift that I would not take for granted. This was exactly the positive experience I needed on my first day as I transitioned into the full-time role of a novice nurse educator teaching students in an academic nursing program.

Although I wish all of my students were as willing to learn as Sun, many were not. Students brought to the learning environment their own values and beliefs about education. Not all of my students valued the experiences that came with education. One example in particular was a student I will call "Lemon" because this student often displayed a negative and "sour" attitude toward learning and faculty. In the afternoon of my first day of teaching, I met Lemon in the nursing skills lab. Throughout the lab practice period, this student had very little positive input to contribute to the learning experience. Lemon challenged my teaching endeavors and occasionally would disrupt the learning environment with unwelcomed humor or irrelevant statements. On this day, I remember Lemon entered the skills lab armed with a negative attitude. Anticipating unwanted disruption to the learning process of other students, I knew that I had to think quickly about how to change the outcome of what I was expecting. I thought that if I allowed Lemon's negative behavior to continue, learning for everyone, especially Lemon, would be affected. For a brief moment, I did not know what to do. I found myself in new territory in an unfamiliar situation. I had never been the primary educator for nursing students before, and had certainly never had to address a student's uncivil behavior. I started to wonder whether I had made the right decision to move into teaching instead of staying in my familiar clinical territory. After much contemplation, I spoke with Lemon about my observation of her behavior. I would like to say that Lemon's behavior changed instantaneously, but the truth is, it did not. It took time to simply scratch the surface of this student's behavior. Each time I taught the nursing skills lab and witnessed her behavior, I felt like a failure as a teacher. I was worried that I had stumbled upon a person whom I would not be able to help through education.

Clinical Teaching

My first clinical day experience was a bit more intense. Yes, I was very excited to take students into the clinical setting. As an experienced clinician and former preceptor for student nurses, the clinical setting was familiar territory for me. However, I had grown accustomed to only having to take the responsibility for two or three students at one time, not 10. Just as I had done on my first day in the classroom, I started to struggle within myself about my ability to function effectively in the role of a clinical educator.

At 6:00 a.m., I arrived at my assigned clinical site, a long-term care facility, greeted the nursing staff, and made student assignments. My confidence level was high; I was organized and armed with a well thought-out agenda for the day. I was ready for my students to come through the door in their pristine nursing uniforms with their skills lab kit in hand, ready to demonstrate safe patient-care nursing skills, and they did. Well, some of them did. As my students started to trickle in at 6:30 a.m., I could feel my calmness disappearing because of the number of students I had to guide alone. I wish I could say that the feeling of insecurity went away quickly, but it did not. However, I was able to manage without students recognizing just how nervous I really was.

After redirecting my thoughts toward my students and not my insecurities, I facilitated a morning briefing with my students. I provided students with a copy of the daily plan, reiterated clinical expectations, shared a brief nurse report, made patient assignments, and most importantly asked students if they had any fears about the day. Yes, I never forgot the lesson Lauren had taught me. With the formalities of the morning addressed, my students headed out to greet their patients and perform basic clinical nursing skills under my direct supervision. To my surprise, once the students met their assigned patients, most of them appeared to be relaxed and confident. Some were able to demonstrate, with accuracy, implementation of their basic nursing skills, such as bed baths, physical assessments, medication administrations, oral and tube feeding, wound care dressing changes, patient teaching, and chart documentation.

I must admit that it was very challenging to keep eyes on all 10 students at the same time and to be with each one of them at the same time. Identifying this challenge early on in the 8-hour shift, I asked the nursing staff at the facility to share in the outcome of my students' learning experiences by helping me to oversee them while they were in the facility. I found that this partnership worked well because it allowed the staff to indirectly contribute to the students' learning process, which several of the nurses had wanted to do.

A second challenge I faced on the first clinical day was learning how to work with multiple students at their different individual levels of comfort and confidence. I had some students that were assertive and excited and ready to tackle any skill opportunity that came their way. Then, I had those that I had to spend extra time with to encourage and reassure that they could perform the task before them. Again, this was unfamiliar territory for me at the student level but I reflected back on my clinician experiences of teaching patients and their families and used those strategies to guide my students. To my surprise, it worked. Though not all of my students were able to show strong confidence in their performance abilities on the first day of clinical, more than half of them were. This made me very proud as a new clinical nurse educator.

In essence, my first clinical day consisted of literally 8 hours of speed walking up and down unit hallways and in and out of patients' rooms coordinating, demonstrating, facilitating, and supervising the clinical learning opportunities of all 10 of my students. At times, I also found myself in the roles of a motivational coach and a comforter for teary-eyed students. At the end of a long first clinical day, I found myself to be mentally and physically exhausted, but at the same time overwhelmingly proud of the clinical experiences I had provided for my students. Prior to leaving the facility, my students expressed how they were satisfied with their clinical experiences and performances for the day. They shared how they took pride in knowing that their patients had been fed and were clean and dry. They also were able to witness their patients exchanging smiles while sitting up in their wheelchairs chatting with other patients, or simply lying in bed while visiting with family members. Nursing staff also gave kudos to how well the day had gone and how my students had performed such great patient care.

At the end of my first day, I experienced a plethora of emotions. Fear crept in when I thought about my lack of experience with teaching students but faded as I realized that even as a novice clinical nurse educator, I was able to draw from my past experiences to problem solve. All of my clinical experiences were valuable and foundational to my success as a novice nurse educator. I was prepared to function in the role, whether in the classroom, lab, or clinical setting. I had survived my first day of teaching students!

RESOURCES NEEDED

As I continued my journey of transitioning from a clinician into a nurse educator role, I realized that having the proper resources, support, and guidance in the learning environment was essential to my ability to teach students effectively and students' ability to be academically successful. It was important to me that I had the support of my nursing director, semester coordinator, and colleagues. This played a significant role in my transition to becoming a nurse educator. My nursing director ensured access for me to continuing education training specific to nurse educators, and authorized me time to actively participate in those programs. My semester coordinator provided me guidance and mentorship through the process of informal transmission of wisdom, relevant knowledge, and shared teaching experiences. Through this relationship, I learned about effective and ineffective teaching strategies. The support and encouragement of my colleagues also helped build my confidence. Experiencing the spirit of a team helped me to maintain a positive outlook on my new role and encouraged me to keep coming back every day. To date, I still find myself collaborating with these three groups of people to seek their advice, leadership, and wisdom. However, I tend to communicate and seek out most of my support needs from my mentor.

From my perspective, mentorship is essential to the new nurse educator. The mentorship support I received initially empowered me with information, opportunities, and experiences as a nurse educator. These elements developed and enhanced my teaching. I gained useful insight into the role of a nurse educator and learned specific skills and knowledge relevant to an effective teaching and learning environment. Another important aspect I gathered from my mentorship experience was knowledge about the organization's culture and unspoken rules, which became critical to my own success as a nurse educator. My mentor provided critical feedback in key areas such as communication, interpersonal relationships, teaching abilities, change management, and leadership skills, and related each one to my nurse educator role. With each year of teaching, I have found that the wisdom and experiences shared with me at the beginning of my nurse educator journey has been foundational to the nurse educator I am today. Although I may no longer require my mentor to be on speed dial, I still have the need to call her occasionally when unfamiliar circumstances in the teaching environment surface or when personal or professional decisions arise. I believe that despite one's years of teaching experiences, the desire and sense of need for mentorship never disappear.

Having the support of my nurse administrator, mentor, and colleagues was important to my success as a nurse educator, but I also needed continuing professional development in order to keep abreast of the frequent theoretical and technical changes that occur in nursing. As a clinician I realized that working in the acute care setting allowed me to work closely with multidisciplinary health care teams, which made me more aware of changes occurring in patient care. However, as a nurse educator, I primarily focused on my one or two assigned courses and became less aware of changes occurring in different aspects of nursing. Having access and time to attend continuing professional development programs remain essential in my educator role.

Continuing professional development has also helped me learn how to design curricula, develop nursing courses, teach effectively, evaluate learning, and document educational outcomes. In addition, professional development has prepared me to advise students, engage in scholarly work, participate in professional associations, present at nursing conferences, and write grant proposals. In essence, I have been taught the full scope of the educator role through these continuing education opportunities.

THE NURSE EDUCATOR ROLE

One thing I love about my role as a nurse educator is that every day is a new adventure. No two days are the same, even when I try to establish a routine. A typical day for me consists of preparing students' learning activities, facilitating students' classroom and clinical learning experiences, counseling and advising students, chairing committee meetings, attending leadership meetings, acknowledging colleagues, and juggling administrative duties. For example, prior to reaching my office from the parking lot, I generally run into one or two students requesting to see me before class starts at 9 o'clock. Most often I agree to see each student right away, which means I have to rush into my office, turn on my computer, and usher them in. Depending on the needs of the student, I may conduct a quick exam review, demonstrate how to work a math problem, reiterate a previously lectured concept, complete and/or sign a form or two, or simply become a pair of listening ears resulting in some form of counseling or advising.

By now, a minimum of 15 or 20 minutes of my 1-hour class prep time has gone by and I am scrambling to listen to phone messages left from the evening before and check my work e-mails to see if any impromptu meeting has been scheduled for the day or if there are urgent messages needing to be addressed right away. During this time I am also acknowledging greetings, questions, or concerns from my colleagues as they individually pass my office door, or stop and trickle in for small talk.

With about 15 minutes before it is time for my class to start, I hurriedly gather my teaching supplies and race from the second floor to the first floor where students noisily await my arrival to the classroom. I then prepare students for the learning process by sharing with them the learning objectives, activities, and expected outcomes for the day. After an hour and a half of facilitating students' learning experiences, I stay after class an extra 10 to 15 minutes to address any questions students may have. Once I have completed my classroom or lab time with students for the day, I return to my office for a short break and then scurry to the first of at least two to three scheduled meetings, and one impromptu meeting for the day. In between meetings, I continue to address the needs of my students as they arise, assist colleagues as needed, prepare for the next work day, and complete additional administrative and committee duties as assigned.

Throughout the day as I juggle multiple administrative tasks and work with students, I sometimes wonder, with all my responsibilities as nurse educator, whether I am as effective for students as I need to be. I think about whether or not I am explaining concepts in a culturally diverse manner that meets the individual needs of all my students. I also wonder to what extent my areas of inexperience as a nurse educator influences my students' learning outcomes. After I advise students and they leave my office, I think about if I really got through to them or should I have immediately sent them to a more experienced faculty member. At the end of each workday, there are many "What if?" and "Should I have?" questions that race through my mind. Some days I leave work feeling like I have led students down the path of success, but then there are other days when I question whether or not I fit the mold of a true nurse educator. Each day brings with it highs and lows. Days that I experience the lows, I find comfort in knowing that I provided students with my best for that day because I took the time to prepare myself to develop and facilitate a positive learning opportunity for them.

To prepare for teaching, I review my daily plan as well as the objectives and goals for the day. I then prioritize other job-related tasks based on the level of importance and the need for immediate attention versus those tasks that can wait. I review my teaching materials once again before entering the class or lab to ensure I did not leave out a concept or skill that I want the students to learn for the day. I take the time to make sure my teaching objectives are purposeful and aligned with the class learning activities for the content being taught. This helps me to ensure that the outcome(s) I want students to achieve from the lesson are obtainable. If I am going to lecture, I practice speaking my presentation out loud, which helps me to re-familiarize myself with the content.

Another aspect of my preparation for the day is making sure I have developed appropriate assignments for students. When making assignments for students, I consider students' knowledge levels about the focused topic or skill and how the assignment promotes students' professional growth. I also consider students' learning styles and the teaching approaches that best meet the various styles. I try to design assignments that are reasonable in difficulty and time so students are not burdened with excessive or unnecessary work.

To assess whether or not students met the intended learning objectives and goals for the day, appropriate evaluation methods are considered. When evaluating students, I consider if the evaluation tool was prepared to address each of the learning outcomes and if the evaluation tool or process was objective and fair. However, I also shift some of the evaluation results on the students by considering if they came prepared or not to meet the learning objectives. For example, I consider students' attendance pattern, if they review the topic materials prior to coming to the learning environment, and if they present with a willingness and readiness to learn. Student information gathered through the evaluation process helps me determine which teaching style and teaching strategies are most effective in achieving the desired learning outcomes.

My personal teaching style is that of a facilitator, though occasionally I may choose to use a delegator, demonstrator, or blended (hybrid) style approach depending upon my student audience and the learning content. With regard to teaching strategies, I aim to be versatile in my approach. Examples of teaching strategies I use to facilitate student learning include lecturing; active learning activities (e.g., hands-on skill practice, role play, and simulation scenarios); cooperative learning (e.g., small group projects and group discussion); technology integration (e.g., online assignments); and case-based teaching (e.g., case studies). Regardless of the teaching strategies I select to implement with students in the learning environment, my overall goal is to use methodologies that engage students in the learning process and help them develop critical thinking skills.

However, I have learned that choosing the correct teaching strategy may not always be possible, thus causing unwarranted student challenges in the learning environment. For example, in an attempt to teach a topic on cardiovascular disease to a new cohort of level one nursing students, I presented the information using a style of teaching I do not use often, the lecture style. I found that if I lecture only, students tend to sit passively, appearing to be listening, but contribute very little to the active learning process. Because of the complexity of the topic, I thought this would be the best method of content delivery. However, approximately 1 week later, through students' test exam results, I found that greater than 50% of the student cohort failed the exam. I quickly realized that the lecture style was not suitable for a complex topic like cardiovascular disease for this group of students. This incident challenged me to reevaluate my teaching method. In an effort to rectify the problem, through an open forum, I evaluated the students' perception of how they felt they could learn the cardiovascular content best. I found that these students preferred to learn about the function of the heart in an active learning environment using high-fidelity simulation manikins in conjunction with brief explanations of major cardiovascular concepts. As a result of changing my teaching method from passive to active, these students were able to retest on the cardiovascular content and greater than 95% of the cohort successfully passed the exam. These students were also able to demonstrate competency of the cardiovascular concepts through skills application in the simulation lab. I feel I was able to make a difference in the learning success of my students just by listening to them and providing a more suitable learning environment for them.

LESSONS LEARNED FROM TRANSITIONING TO THE NURSE EDUCATOR ROLE

Despite my successes as a nurse educator, I know that there is much for me to learn. In striving to grow and develop into the most effective nurse educator I can be for my students, I continue to pursue education for myself. Over the last 4 years I studied hard and worked tirelessly to satisfy the requirements of a doctor of education degree. The knowledge and experiences gathered through the work toward this advanced level of education, coupled with my previous formal nursing education and clinical experiences, have certainly helped to prepare me for transitioning from a clinical expert to the nurse educator role. However, I am well aware that education alone cannot help a clinician effectively transition into this role and that additional preparation is needed.

It has taken a team approach to help transition me into the nurse educator I am today. I needed the support of my administrator, mentor, and colleagues as well and the organization I left. Maintaining a supportive collaborative relationship with my clinical family in my previous positions was essential to my transition because it allowed me to embrace the changes in my new role without regrets or hesitations. The most important factor that has influenced my decision to remain in the nurse educator role is my ability to play the integral part in the nursing profession that I had always hoped. I have been able to achieve what I consider to be my greatest contribution to nursing, which is to help others help themselves through education, by teaching them to think critically and intensively and to develop professional character.

I have learned that as a nurse educator you must have deep passion for inspiring others to be better and to do better through the power of education. For a new nurse educator, though the passion to teach may lay deep within the soul and the intent is to become an effective educator, both can easily be trampled down by the challenges that come with the role. Based on my transitional experiences from the role of an expert clinician to one of a novice nurse educator, I think it is necessary for educational programs and clinical sites to facilitate the role of a new nurse educator. To do this, I suggest that new nurse educators be shown support, understanding, and patience from both their departing and accepting administrations. They also need to be provided with professional development and mentorships specific to the role of a nurse educator. Finally, as a transitioning nurse educator, I would suggest that educational programs and clinical sites consider this one thought when facilitating the role of a new educator:

> *Let us think of education as a means of developing our greatest abilities, because in each of us there is a private hope and dream which, fulfilled, can be translated into benefit for everyone and greater strength for our nation.*
>
> —John F. Kennedy

CHAPTER 9

Reflections of a Clinical Educator in a Hospital Setting

Meggen Platzar

The mediocre teacher tells. The good teacher explains. The superior teacher demonstrates. The great teacher inspires.

—William Arthur Ward

This quote is hanging on a wall in my work cubicle to serve as a reminder why I became a nurse and why I want to be a nurse educator. As soon as I became a nurse, I also became an educator. I believe all nurses are educators because we help our patients and our fellow coworkers by constantly collecting and sharing knowledge. We quickly learn that in the world of nursing practice, knowledge must be shared.

I was a blank slate when I entered the field of nursing. I did not know anyone who was a nurse and did not have an accurate depiction of what a nurse did. My original desire to become a nurse stemmed from my experiences surrounding the birth of my son. I observed my labor and delivery nurse start my IV, hang my IV fluids, titrate my drips, and provide my husband and me with emotional support. I was so inspired by her intelligence and compassion that I myself became inspired to pursue a nursing career. As I reflect on this time, I cannot think of a higher honor anyone can achieve than to inspire another into his or her chosen field. I wanted to do my part and make my mark on humanity.

Shortly after the birth of my son, I started nursing school. My studies were challenging and rewarding. I worked as a nurse's assistant in a long-term care facility during my second year of school. I chose this setting because I felt a connection with the geriatric population because of visiting my great-grandmother in her facility. However, I quickly learned that the long-term care setting, as opposed to acute care, was not my passion and so this became a short-lived job. I spent the rest of the time waitressing through college. My clinicals were where I obtained the majority of my exposure to the inpatient culture. I instantly loved the environment.

After graduating from nursing school, I only wanted to work at one hospital—the Cleveland Clinic. I started on an inpatient internal medicine unit. I had completed several clinicals there and was amazed at the complexity of patients, as well as the skill of the nurses. I felt a sense of pride and commitment to the organization and the nursing profession. For the first time in my short span of life, I felt like a true professional.

My early experiences in an RN role largely influenced my later career choice to become a nurse educator. This started during my orientation, which was accompanied by many positives and some negatives. The positive characteristics of my orientation were made possible by a preceptor who was strong clinically, adhered to policy strictly, and advocated for patients. I learned so much simply by role modeling these behaviors in my own practice. The orientation program was strong and guided by clinical instructors who touched base with us frequently in casual meetings; so, by the end of my 12 weeks, I had a manager and coach telling me that I was ready to practice without a preceptor.

What would we learn if we just focused on the strengths of programs and not the opportunities for improvement? This orientation period seemed pretty typical, but I found myself feeling alone and isolated in my feelings of anxiety. What if I make a mistake? What if I cause harm to a patient? What if the staff does not like me? People tell me I am doing a good job, but what does "good" mean? A lot of this anxiety was due, in large part, to the "watch one, do one" mentality. I was left to do a lot of things on my own and was expected to know when to come and get someone if I needed help. However, I was looking for more direction and support and wanted to be "coached" as I was completing tasks. I did not want to share my anxieties with anyone because I did not want them to think that I could not handle the workload. I spent a lot of time talking to my husband, who was trying hard to understand my medical lingo. This did not ease my anxieties. To make matters worse, I had missed a mandatory class that I was supposed to attend. My manager reprimanded me at the nurses' station in front of my colleagues. This small act diminished my confidence and I looked at my manager as someone whom I should avoid at all costs lest she find more inadequacies in me. Right there, I had lost another resource. All of this anxiety became amplified once I was out of orientation. I was wondering if I had what it took to be a nurse, if I was intelligent enough, strong enough, and assertive enough. I wondered if I was completely insane for wanting to get into a field that came with such high stakes.

As time passed, I got past my initial anxiety and actually started to enjoy the art of nursing. I was getting positive feedback from patients. I was handling a variety of clinical situations on the medical unit. I kept hearing people say that my unit was a "great unit to start out on." I would look back and agree with everyone. I dealt with patients who had everything from chest pain and sepsis, to multiple sclerosis and sickle cell anemia. My clinical knowledge exploded within a year and I started to feel more confident.

After orientation, I was encouraged to further my clinical knowledge with education. I became ACLS (Advanced Cardiovascular Life Support) certified and took skin care classes, all of which helped boost my confidence. I was asked to be a "champion" for our unit's conversion to electronic documentation. I felt honored and valued as a team member.

DECISION TO BECOME A NURSE EDUCATOR

My decision to leave the clinical unit and become a nurse educator was an easy one. I felt like I was born to fulfill the educator role. Unbeknownst to me, my journey toward becoming a nurse educator started when I was asked to become a preceptor for a new nurse graduate. I immediately said, "Yes! I would love to do it!" I think I reacted to the simple fact that I was shocked I was even asked. I took this as a sign that in my own short time in clinical practice, I had shown growth and competence and my leadership team wanted me to share my skills with a new staff member. I later found out that sometimes this is not the case. Preceptors were sometimes asked to mentor simply because there was no one else to do it. Regardless of the reason, I felt extremely honored. Soon, however, my quickness to respond was replaced with feelings of doubt because I still felt new myself. It was at this point that the enormity of the job started to sink in. However, this time, instead of fear, I felt an extreme sense of responsibility to teach this nurse everything she needed to know on how to be successful. I felt like her success as an RN was a testament to my success as a preceptor.

My first precepting experience came with some unexpected rewards. I found a style of education that worked for myself and the RN that I was precepting. I found that questioning her, and allowing her to come up with the answers, helped me to understand her thought processes. At the same time, this helped build her self-confidence. I felt like I was off to a great start as a preceptor because I was able to instill confidence in this new RN. The relationship we built as colleagues was important and I ended up gaining a lifelong friend. I did not just teach her skills and protocols, but I also mentored her. I became a mentor in the sense that I taught her about hospital culture, dealing with patient and family emotions, dealing with difficult staff members, and helping her through the rough new period where she felt she was incompetent. I felt like I had the opportunity to make a positive impact on someone else's career. I am not sure how she feels looking back on her orientation experience, but I hope that I had a positive impact on her practice. After this experience, I had the honor of orienting many other nurses. Each precepting relationship was unique, yet the same teaching/ facilitation principles applied.

Through functioning as a preceptor, I had the opportunity to work closely with our unit-based clinical instructor. The clinical instructor role intrigued and inspired me because it blended clinical nursing and education. It expanded my horizons and provided a different perspective about another nursing role. Our unit-based clinical instructor had hinted several times that she felt I would perform well in her role. She herself was leaving the department and was trying to recruit people in whom she saw potential. I wanted to apply for the role, but at the time, I only had my associate's degree. This event was a big factor in my pursuit of a bachelor's degree in nursing.

When I finally graduated with my bachelor's, an opportunity within our nursing education department opened up. I applied and obtained the position. Walking into the interview, I felt very prepared to take on any assignment or expectation they would throw my way. I had a few years under my belt, had served on multiple committees, and was the primary preceptor for many nurses. I felt ready! However, as the interview progressed, there was a part of me that was becoming slightly apprehensive. The hospital-based clinical instructors were responsible for unit-based in-servicing for many inpatient units, coordinating the orientations of new staff members, responding to rapid responses, codes, CITs [crisis intervention related to a hostile patient], attending department meetings, teaching orientation classes, EKG classes, BLS, ACLS, hospital-based initiatives, participating on committees, and in the end, becoming the expert nurse on their units. My head was spinning on how I could accomplish all that in a 40-hour work week. After reviewing the list of responsibilities, I was concerned that I did not "know enough" to educate colleagues and mentor new nurses. However, I had felt this feeling before and this time, I was much better equipped to deal with it.

STARTING AS A NURSE EDUCATOR

I will never forget my level of anticipation on my first day as a formal nurse educator. Even though the likelihood of me having to educate anyone on the first day was slim to none, I was nervous about starting on this new adventure. This, to me, was like starting a whole new career. I wanted to prove to my new supervisor and coworkers that I had what it took to be an educator. I started by observing my preceptor teaching an in-service for one unit's night shift staff that was based on a request of the manager and staff. I could not wait to do the same for my units. My preceptor was planning on flexing her hours that day so she started at 6:00 a.m. for the in-service and planned to leave at 3:00 p.m. As simple as this flextime sounds, this was a new concept for me since my life as a bedside nurse had been so structured. I found flextime to be extremely professional in the sense that I was trusted to manage my time while still completing all the work I needed to do.

After the in-service, my preceptor took me to the units I would be covering and introduced me to some of the nurses and managers. Shortly afterward, we headed to a meeting that the hospital-wide clinical instructors, clinical nurse specialists, and nursing informatics team attended. The purpose of the meeting was to address the recent changes that were made to our electronic documentation workflow. The discussion was centered on what education plan existed to introduce the new workflow to our nurses. Some of the discussion also focused on the applicability and user friendliness of the system. The discussion was professional and assertive. Each member of the staff stated his or her viewpoint with an admirable linguistic precision that reflected deep thought and inquisitive intelligence. I was impressed by the ability of the members to articulate their thoughts so well. I felt proud to be part of such an impressive group. However, the greatest impression this meeting left on me was just how far nursing education extended. My department was not simply about teaching someone how to insert an IV, teaching a class, or even helping a new nurse successfully transition to practice. Its influence reached into every aspect, every possible corner of nursing practice. Rolling out new electronic software? How are we going to teach the nurses? How are we going to guarantee high compliance? It was incredible to think about all the ways nursing education tied everything together with the bedside nurse always being at the forefront.

Fortunately, my preceptor and I developed a healthy professional relationship. I noticed that her role was different from my view of a traditional preceptor in the sense that my orientation period was very autonomous. She was there to provide resources if needed and to assist in decision making, but she was not there to make decisions for me. As much as I appreciated this orientation model, at the same time I still felt unprepared in my role as an educator. I had to adjust to the autonomy of my role. Instead of my day being directed by patient activities, it was now directed by the nurse caring for the patient. To decide where I should be focusing my time, I needed to find out what the nurses needed.

To begin, I set up meetings with the nurse managers and other members of the management teams. The meeting involved, first and foremost, getting to know them and understanding their leadership styles. It also was important to understand their expectations of me. This crucial conversation provided an open dialogue in which roles and goals could be established and a relationship of trust could begin to be built. Next, I met with the nurses by rounding on the units and sending out contact information. Upon reflection, it might have been better to send formal introduction letters to the nurses, as well as hosting focus groups. This may have helped me more quickly build rapport and establish credibility. The next item on my agenda was to acquaint myself with the patient populations. I accomplished this by shadowing nurses and working a shift on the unit. Looking back, I wish I had spent more time working on the floor. I needed much more prep than a single shift, even though I had worked with some of the populations previously. Finally, the part that ties this all together is that I had to understand the culture of the units I was serving. I accomplished this by completing all three of the previously stated interventions and then documenting my thoughts and observations. Reviewing these observations gave me insight into structured processes, time management, and teamwork on the unit.

Another helpful tool that the department as a whole used was an education survey. This tool provides information about the workforce mixture, requested in-services, preferred education style, and time of day nurses were most willing to attend an educational activity. This survey helped create the education profile for the unit. It also served as a useful tool in ensuring accurate communication with managers about their units' education needs. All of these tasks on my agenda helped me reach my goal of becoming a valuable resource for my units.

Thankfully, in my career as a clinical educator, I have had the pleasure of experiencing those same positive feelings I received while precepting new nurses. One such experience occurred after I had taught a relatively new class to a group of my nursing peers with whom I had worked as a bedside nurse. I had the greatest respect for these nurses who helped shape me into the nurse I am today. One of the more senior nurses told me that was one of the best classes she had attended. She said that it seemed to her that I was born to teach. This positive feedback was invaluable; in this moment, I truly felt that I was making a difference.

Another positive experience occurred while I was helping a new graduate nurse during orientation. The nurse became very sick and needed to be hospitalized. Despite her ill health, she was concerned about missing work and classes that she knew were mandatory. Overcome with feelings of sympathy for the position my new nurse was in, I visited her in the hospital and tried to put her mind at ease in regard to the classes and shifts she was missing. She expressed gratitude for the comfort. I felt extremely helpless for this new nurse, who was trying not only to keep up with all of her onboarding responsibilities, but also to maintain her health. I forged a strong relationship with that nurse and she forever will be a part of my positive experiences as a new clinical nurse educator. This act and other acts were observed by some of my colleagues and they nominated me for an award I received later that year. There is no greater compliment than to be recognized for your hard work and commitment by your peers.

CHALLENGES AS A NEW NURSE EDUCATOR

With every new experience in life, one must appreciate the positives and negatives, although in time, we come to see the negatives as stepping stones of progress. The negatives develop into challenges that give us the opportunity to improve our practice and ourselves as human beings.

I have had my fair share of challenges in my role. One that comes to mind is the first time I taught an EKG class with my preceptor. This was day 2 of the EKG class and the students were expected to have already built basics upon a small foundation of knowledge in the first class. We were not planning on teaching this particular class on that day, but were asked to pick up the class by another educator who had a family emergency. Wanting to help out a coworker in her time of need, my preceptor agreed to teach the class for her. When we started going through the material in the class, the nurses had several questions, some basic, some very complicated. I immediately was intimidated by the sheer volume of questions and the number of people in the class. There were approximately 40 students and I had never taught a class that large before. Since I was still trying to adjust to my new role as an educator, I was not able to answer all of the questions. I felt fortunate that my preceptor could answer most. I was afraid of teaching a class and seeming like I did not know what I was talking about. I vowed that, from that day on, I was going to do everything I could to prepare for any class I was going to teach.

As I gained more experience as an educator, my apprehensiveness has drastically decreased; however, whenever I am planning something new, all of those anxieties come back, perhaps not as strong, but still there. For instance, the first time I presented at a nursing conference, I had large butterflies fluttering around in my stomach. This feeling has always been a way for me to harness nervous energy into the production of a great product. In this case, that product was a presentation. I have also noticed that my comfort level with my leadership abilities has increased. This has helped me achieve a comfort level with my learners and coworkers. Although I now feel that I am comfortable in my role,

I am just not always comfortable with what I am teaching. Health care is always evolving and our policies are ever changing. All of this helps me strive to be at the forefront of new information. How can an instructor be influential, affect practice, and be an invaluable resource if he or she is out of touch with the newest policies? I feel that would send a message that stagnation is acceptable, and that simply is not the case.

RESOURCES NEEDED

Knowledge and availability of resources is what helps to make a good unit-based clinical instructor. At the same time, for many leadership positions, the ability to network and support staff is very important. When starting my career as a nursing educator, support from my peers within my department was vital to my successful transition. Their support helped me with personal growth and understanding of my role, but they also were important resources to my staff. In supporting each other in our educator roles, we would review PowerPoints prior to one of us presenting, or we would plan a mock presentation in a meeting room with a handful of peers and critique presenting styles. Having these types of resources helped me grow as an educator. The staff helped keep the bar high within our department. Even after my educator orientation, many questions arose on a daily basis. These could range from the simple, "Who can I borrow a manikin from?" to the more complex, "What changes were made to the central line policy?" Just as we tell our new nurses to use their resources, such as their managers and charge nurses, so should new educators use their resources of experts in their departments. My educator colleagues and I also work closely with our clinical nurse specialists and function as a highly effective team. We help each other teach in-services and share material we have already developed. In this way, we have all become better educators.

Another important resource is the nurse manager. It is vitally important to establish a professional relationship with the nurse managers. When communication lines are open, managers will express the learning needs of their staff and facilitate a better understanding of how the educator can maximize results. If the communication is poor, scope creep may ensue so that the educator feels he or she is being pulled to do things that do not fit under his or her role. Scope creep can become overwhelming and leave one with feelings of inadequacy.

Another important resource is knowledge of the nursing staff, who are the eyes and ears of the unit and will communicate frequently about education needs, progress of a new nurse, or incidents that have occurred on the unit. A clinical educator's first and foremost priority is to support the nursing staff in their ability to provide high-quality patient care.

There are always resources available that not all people take advantage of; one of those resources is mentorship. It is an important part of any leadership role because it provides the key to the door of experience and knowledge. When I first started as an educator, I did not take advantage of this resource. There were many things for which I needed career advice, including how to better manage my time, how to better communicate to a mass audience, how to show discretion when deciding educational classes/in-services, how to work online education programs, and how to maximize my strengths and work on my areas needing improvement. Despite my support within the department, a mentor who had more experience and a professional career that I admired could have made an impact on my early career decisions.

Now a couple of years into my educator role, I have acquired two mentors. My first mentor is my immediate supervisor. A typical mentor is often not one's supervisor, but is easily accessible and invested in one's growth. My supervisor has provided me with sound career advice and supports me in decision making. My second mentor I acquired through a leadership development program. She does not work in nursing education and I find that having a mentor who is not within my department is just as helpful as having one who is. She has given me access to a number of useful tools to help me get organized, as well as pointers on having crucial conversations. As I move forward with my career, and if I ever switch departments, I will seek out a mentor right from the beginning.

Finally, I want to mention the importance of ongoing education for educators. I recently had the pleasure of attending a yearlong leadership training program that included classroom, online, and field education. Some of the classes I attended included such strategies as improving presentation skills, including how to make a great presentation and the power of body language while teaching, coaching, project management, and leadership presence. My thirst to develop professionally while I developed others was being quenched. I think the role of the educator in the hospital setting is an ever-evolving one and therefore may not be well defined. It is important to take advantage of all resources offered and mold the role into something powerful and influential.

THE NURSE EDUCATOR ROLE

My typical day as a nurse educator has changed quite a bit since I began. Our nursing education department has experienced an immense amount of change in the last 4 years. In my first year, we changed the entire way we framed nursing orientation. We adopted a testing tool that would give us an opportunity to assess our new hire nurses' ability to think critically and then pinpoint their strengths and opportunities for growth. This information is then used to format and individualize their orientation. I have also experienced a series of changes of direct supervisors, directors, unit mangers, and units covered. Born from this change were several exciting new programs for our new nurse graduates. One of those was the formation of a new nurse residency program.

The nurse residency program consists of a strong core curriculum and competency standards. Our residents spend varying lengths of time in orientation based on their test results and clinical competence. After their initial orientation period, they are required to come back for residency education on days that are spread out throughout their first year of hire. One of the new roles that emerged from the residency program was the creation of our Enterprise Residency Support (ERS) team. This is a team of six educators who follow all newly graduated nurse residents in each of the hospitals in our health system. The chance to participate in something new and groundbreaking was irresistible, so I accepted the role of leading this small team of educators.

Our team's expectations include coordinating orientation by meeting with the residents up to five times within a 10-week period. Each of these meetings has a standard form that needs to be filled out and is designed to identify whether they are meeting, exceeding, or not reaching the expectations of the core curriculum. By the end of 2014, our team had worked with over 538 nurse residents. This is by far the most important role of the team. On any given day, I could visit three different hospitals and see up to seven different nurse residents. The meetings typically last around an hour and we strongly encourage the coach and a member of the management team to attend. Each meeting is set up to use artful questioning to determine the level of critical thinking the nurses have developed. Having them describe their patient load and talk about their patients' situations, backgrounds, assessments, and recommended interventions provides an excellent perspective into their ability to understand the patient picture. I have learned that if the nurse resident is not the one speaking during most of the meeting, then it was not a very good meeting. Since I essentially am trying to assess their abilities and help them come up with the answers, they should be directing the meeting content. The team also sets up touch points with the nurse residents after their initial orientation period. These occur on the residency education days, and on 6-month and 1-year anniversaries.

One of the challenges I face on a day-to-day basis is ensuring that the nurses are meeting the requirements of the core curriculum. When there is an obvious problem, such as a lack of critical thinking demonstrated by the nurse, immediate interventions must be taken to help that nurse get up to speed quickly. The challenge lies in identifying the cause of the lack of critical thinking. Is it an issue specifically with knowledge deficit? Is it due to lack of the nurse's initiative? Is the coach being ineffective? Depending on what the issue is, the correct intervention must follow. Not identifying the correct problem will make an intervention unsuccessful no matter how hard we try. Delaying identification can have a poor impact on that nurse's orientation and may impact patient care. I continue to build on my skill of identifying learning deficits and initiating education plans.

Our second vital role is supporting the nurse resident's coach. We use the term "coach" instead of preceptor to reflect a style of education to be used with the nurse residents. During our meetings with the nurse residents, we openly encourage the coaches to provide feedback about residents' progress. This provides residents the opportunity to get positive and constructive feedback on a consistent basis, allowing them time to reflect and change practice if needed. We identify that the nurse resident is getting exposure to a variety of patient populations seen on the unit and requests help from the coach to locate different patients and skills to maximize the learning process. Our team, along with educators from our department, has developed coach training. We then facilitate the classes on coach education.

A third role of the ERS team is their engagement in residency education days. We, along with a group of exceptional clinical educators and clinical nurse specialists, helped develop the curriculum for the education days as well as teach these classes. One of the most rewarding parts of these education days is the beginning of the class when our team facilitates discussions with the nurse residents. The topics can range from describing their clinical experiences, to lessons learned that they applied in the clinical setting, to areas where they have ideas for process improvement. The openness and honesty of our nurse residents still impresses me to this day and speaks to the strong relationships formed with the instructors.

Starting something new is always exciting and hard work. My current work weeks can be long, yet productive. My preparation occurs for the whole week instead of day by day, mostly due to the variety of places I visit throughout the week. Time management is critically important. Since my workload changes constantly, it is up to me to find ways to manage my time effectively. Meeting with residents, running effective meetings, and teaching classes are skills I feel I have effectively developed. There is always room for improvement, but I have acquired experience and knowledge that help me effectively complete those tasks. My identified areas for growth include keeping track of resident data and finding ways to visually share those data with the team. Becoming more efficient in computer software programs has become increasingly important for my ability to manage my time and track productivity.

In closing, I feel I make a difference every day in my role in educating future nurses of my organization. I hope that through my coaching and teaching, I can inspire a generation of nurses who are eager to learn and display competent and confident practice. I hope I can inspire another wave of educators. If I can inspire, I know I am reaching the level of educator I want to be.

LESSONS LEARNED FROM TRANSITIONING TO THE NURSE EDUCATOR ROLE

Preparation for the role of an educator is important to one's ability to inspire and engage. It can affect the way you are able to educate and how effective you feel in your role. Do I feel that my previous education prepared me for my role of a nurse educator? In some ways yes, and in some ways no. In my organization, to be considered for the role of the clinical nurse educator, you must have been involved in different professional groups prior to taking on the role. Many of us have been chairs for our shared governance councils, charge nurses, preceptors, and active members of professional organizations, so many of the leadership qualities were already in the making. However, I think that I was not prepared for the project management aspect. Being a project manager of a team of people is very different from planning your own educational activities. Planning, executing, and reviewing a new process while leading a team of people presented me with big challenges. I have a renewed appreciation for our project managers and feel this is a great skill to develop.

One of the factors that has had a big influence on my staying in the clinical educator role is the support I have received from my immediate management team and coworkers. Receiving guidance and feedback from my supervisors has affected my job satisfaction. I know now, if I am not receiving feedback, I need to seek it out. If I am to help others grow and learn, I myself must be an active participant in the process. Establishing professional working relations and the creation of a high functioning team have strengthened my commitment to the education department. The opportunity to participate in new education programs has also influenced my decision to continue my career in our education department. However, perhaps the biggest reason why I stay in education is the same reason I fell in love with it: I enjoy supporting the bedside nurse. Every time I hear, "Oh, yeah, that makes sense now" or "So that is why we do that that way" or "Thanks so much for your help," it feeds the caregiver inside me, spiritually.

Looking forward, I feel it would be useful for institutions to create a nurse educator track to help create a career path for their educators. To start on this track, nurses would be expected to join certain committees, assume leadership roles, and attend leadership classes. Then, after they have fulfilled these requirements, they could apply to become an educator. Creating partnerships with local nursing colleges could also help to build consistency between the nurse's academic and clinical education. In the end, our goal is to inspire, so we ourselves must never stop finding and creating reasons to be inspired.

PART IV

Storied Reflections

CHAPTER 10

Learning From Shared Narratives: Pulling It All Together

If you want a happy ending, that depends, of course,
on where you stop your story.

—Orson Welles, in the *Big Brass Ring* screenplay

Stories have the power to engage our imagination and empathy, helping us to explore ways of knowing and practices of thinking that inform our understanding of the nature of experiences (Diekelmann, 2001, p. 54). The nurse clinicians' stories in this book convey the nature of their unique experiences of moving into the role of clinical nurse educators. Their diverse voices of expertise, colored with the concerns that they needed to address in moving out of their comfort zone, can help us understand the important ways that nurses make a difference in the health care system of today.

As noted in the preface, the current shortage of nurse educators is a serious problem. There is a critical need to prepare more nursing students and new graduate nurses for practice but, in order to do this, the shortage of nurse educators needs to be addressed. Understanding the

experiences of clinicians who have moved through the transitional process can help new novice educators gain confidence in their new role.

Educating Nurses: A Call for Radical Transformation (Benner, Sutphen,
Leonard, & Day, 2010) reported findings from the first national nursing
education study in 30 years, sponsored by The Carnegie Foundation
for the Advancement of Teaching. Researchers explored the strengths
and weaknesses in nursing education and the many challenges faced by
the nursing profession. The authors carried out extensive field research
at a wide variety of nursing schools, as well as a national survey of
teachers and students administered in cooperation with the National
League for Nursing (NLN), the American Association of Colleges
of Nursing (AACN), and the National Student Nurses' Association
(NSNA). This landmark study contained four broad recommendations
for future changes in nursing education. These four recommendations
are described here along with suggested strategies for meeting the recommendations that were described in previous chapters.

1. *Move from a focus on teaching decontextualized knowledge to
an emphasis on teaching for a sense if salience, situated cogni-
tion, and action in particular situations.*

Teaching for a sense of salience means helping students
to make connections between acquiring and using knowledge
(Benner et al., 2010, p. 94). Making connections between content
such as pathophysiology learned in the classroom and caring for
a specific patient does not just happen. Clinical nurse educators
need to consciously implement strategies to make this happen.
Novice students often focus on one thing at a time and specific
tasks and may not "see" the clinical situation as a whole. They
need guidance and experience from their clinical educators to
develop a perceptual grasp of the nature of specific clinical situations (Benner et al., 2010).

Continued situated coaching is needed to help students grasp
the changing dynamics of a clinical situation so that they know what
is important and what is most important to address first. Nurse clinicians possess the expertise needed to help students integrate new
knowledge and skills into a practice context. This is reflected in the
pedagogical moments, the *tact of teaching*, and the Socratic pedagogy
strategies discussed in this book. Strategies that clinical educators
can use to help students contextualize knowledge during their

clinical experiences include the following, which relate to effective clinical evaluation strategies that are discussed in Chapter 4:

- Share clear expectations for students and obtain their individual goals for learning.
- Provide frequent opportunities for formative evaluation.
- Work collaboratively with nursing staff on the unit to ensure they are aware of your goals for the students.
- Consult with experienced educators to help you in difficult pass/fail decisions.
- Use clinical journals to provide opportunities for open dialogue between you and the student.
- Consider ways to use high- or low-fidelity simulation as a nonthreatening platform for practicing clinical skills and fostering self-reflection on performance.
- Use multiple sources for gathering data about student performance, such as observation, discussion with staff, and document review.

2. *Integrate clinical and classroom teaching.*

Benner and colleagues (2010), when they visited schools across the country as a part of their research, found a distinct divide between classroom and clinical teaching. For example, students learned skills, such as taking a blood pressure, on healthy volunteers in a decontextualized situation, which was very different from the experience of taking a blood pressure while assessing an anxious and very ill hypertensive patient in the hospital. It is important to identify ways to bridge this gap in know/do learning.

Nurse educators who are teaching in both the clinical area and classroom can plan their classroom teaching activities to extend into the clinical arena, helping students to understand the application of classroom knowledge in diverse clinical situations. This is more difficult for nurse educators who are only in the clinical area. Thus, it is important for classroom and clinical instructors to structure opportunities to share important information for helping students integrate classroom and clinical knowledge and skills. Scheduling meetings with part-time clinical instructors at times that fit their schedules, including telephone or online SKYPE meetings, is helpful in keeping them abreast of classroom objectives and outcomes. Strategies discussed in Chapter 2 for making a difference for students can help them integrate classroom and clinical knowledge:

- Capitalize on the pedagogical moment.
- See the pedagogical possibilities in ordinary incidents.
- Share your own clinical experiences with students.
- Use a variety of teaching/learning strategies to accomplish the course objectives.
- Assign challenging patients—just be there to assist your student, if needed.
- Relate what the students are seeing in the clinical setting with what they are learning in the classroom. Know the curriculum in the school where you teach so you can do this.
- Do not be afraid to ask questions of the full-time faculty or clinical coordinator. They are there to mentor you and assist you in learning about the school, teaching in academia, and the specific objectives of the course you are teaching. Keep their phone numbers/e-mail addresses handy.
- Listen to the students. What are they yearning to learn? What are they fearful of?
- Reflect on your teaching and clinical experiences—we learn through reflection.

3. *Expand the focus on critical thinking to an emphasis on clinical reasoning and multiple ways of thinking.*

As we discussed in Chapter 6, the term "critical thinking" is often used as a catch-all phrase for the many types of thinking that nurses use in practice (Benner et al., 2010). Benner and colleagues noted that students need multiple ways of thinking to develop the perceptual acuity or clinical imagination needed for professional practice. Clinical reasoning, the ability to reason as a clinical situation changes and take into account the context of the situation, with all of its complexities, is essential for clinical decision making. In addition, clinical imagination is needed, which helps nurses to grasp the nature of patients' changing needs over time.

Chapter 6 described how nurse educators can help to teach multiple ways of thinking to their students. These approaches are excellent strategies for clinical nurse educators, as they can help students integrate classroom knowledge with a variety of clinical situations, building skills in clinical reasoning and clinical imagination. Strategies to help build these thinking skills include the following:

- Be comfortable with silence—don't answer your own questions! Don't change the question (unless it really just wasn't clear). Remember that students are *always* more uncomfortable than you with the silence.

- It can be good sometimes (not always) to let students think about a question before answering. Give them a chance to talk with each other or to do five minutes of writing in response to a question. For instance, they might write in response to the questions: "What did we see in this video of the patient? What surprised or concerned you about what you saw?" Students could then share their responses, and those responses would serve as the starting point of discussion.

- If no student volunteers a response to a question, consider calling on a particular student; if that student does not know, most likely another student will help out and rescue him or her. Ideally, "calling on someone in a non-threatening way tends to activate others who might otherwise remain silent" (Garlikov, n.d.).

- Don't overplan a class session. Have some idea of content or questions to be covered, but let the conversation flow where it seems to want to go; in this way, students are engaged and learning what they are ready and interested to learn.

4. *Emphasize the importance of formation and a sense of identity as a professional.*

Benner and colleagues (2010) used the term "formation" to describe changes in identity and self-understanding that occur when transitioning from a lay person role to a professional. Shulman described nursing as a profession with distinctive features that mirror many attributes of other professions but that also has a singular identity of its own (Benner et al., 2010, p. ix). Shulman also noted that the complexity of the nursing profession is paralleled by the complexity of the contexts in which nurses practice (Benner et al., 2010, p. xi). In most professions, practitioners have control over the pace and specific focus of their work, but nurses often need to attend to many clients at the same time, each of whom needs one-on-one treatment. This can be overwhelming for a student who has learned a new skill in the classroom or clinical lab and then needs to implement it in the clinical environment while multitasking and multithinking. This may be especially challenging for students in accelerated programs who are used to thinking in ways needed for their previous professions and now need to learn to "think like a nurse."

Clinical nurse educators can serve a unique role in helping to shape the development of a student as a professional as they role model what it is like to be a professional practitioner. As novices, students may focus on tasks and skills to be learned in the clinical environment but clinical nurse educators can model for them how these tasks and skills must be integrated into the role of a professional. In the 2010 study by Benner and colleagues, students and faculty often spoke of "a-ha" moments when students suddenly realized what it is to be a nurse, including the moral responsibility of being a nurse. Clinical nurse educators cannot plan these pedagogical moments but they can recognize them and help the students to reflect on the experiential learning that takes place in these situations. The following strategies, discussed in Chapter 3 for creating a caring environment, can help students develop a sense of identity as a professional nurse:

- Listen actively to students to learn their expectations and concerns.
- Convey to students a genuine interest and concern for them as individuals and for their learning needs.
- Provide clear explanations of what you expect from students and encourage their feedback related to these explanations.
- Schedule individual conferences for students to share perspectives on their experiences and discuss problems they have encountered; schedule group conferences to help students learn to give and receive support from peers and faculty.
- Structure opportunities for discussion of experiences related to incivility that the students may have encountered.
- Implement creative clinical assignments, such as weekly journals, to encourage student reflection and sharing of concerns.
- Consider cultural influences with your students that may impact their learning.

- Establish effective working relationships with staff members who interact with your students and encourage them to discuss issues of concern with you.

Finally, it is important to think about why you want to transition to a nurse educator role. Is it because you are tired of your present role and want a change? Do you like to teach or feel you have an affinity for teaching? Do you think that the nurse educator role will give you more prestige? Do you feel that this role will allow you to expand your contributions to nursing? It is important to recognize the reason you want to transition into a new role and then to employ strategies for success in your new role.

The following strategies, discussed in Chapter 1, are important in helping you to transition successfully to the nurse educator role:

- Identify your reasons for deciding to transition to the educator role so that you will know what you hope to gain from the experience.
- Identify the strengths that you bring to the educator role, as well as areas in which you believe you need more guidance.
- Share your ideas and concerns with others in the nurse educator role.
- Find a mentor whose advice you trust.
- Keep a journal that describes your experiences so that you can judge your progress in competence in your new role.

As noted frequently in the preceding chapters, the mentoring relationship is a vital part of transitioning successfully from a clinician to a nurse educator role. The following strategies, discussed in Chapter 5, are important to consider in finding and working with a mentor:

- Identify what you want and need in a mentor.
- Seek out one or more persons who can mentor you. Share with them what you need from them.
- Your mentor does not need to be a nurse. Sometimes there are friends or colleagues in other disciplines who may be very effective mentors for you.
- Make the mentoring relationship a win–win experience for both you and your mentor. Think about how you can make the relationship with your mentor beneficial for him or her, as well as for you.
- Keep a reflective journal that describes your mentoring experiences and share these with your mentor.

FIRST-HAND NARRATIVES OF NOVICE NURSE EDUCATORS, EIGHT YEARS LATER

We have kept in touch with some of the nurse educators who attended the Clinical Nurse Educator Academy and some of them have written us about their 8-year journey to their roles today. We have included a few of their reflections here.

Marian is still teaching but not in a full-time role, as the nurse educator salary is considerably less than her clinical manager role:

> I am a lifelong teacher. I have continued to be a nurse manager, always teaching staff, theory and working on policy and procedure development. I have taught as an adjunct at [two colleges]. My most rewarding moment was working with the second degree students and watching them evolve into caring nurses after coming from a degree in business or engineering. Many of them were scared to death of psych but once they understood the pathology and theory, they had buy-in. Role-play always made it so much simpler as well. It was so gratifying and if I thought, I could teach full time and leave my current position … I would.

Hannah also wrote that she could not accept a full-time position as nurse educator because of the lower salary. It is clear, however, that she is still contributing a great deal to education of her colleagues in the clinical area:

> I stayed in nursing administration. I did not go into an educator position. The pay difference was too steep. Now having stated that, I do feel I use my degree all the time. I serve on the Professional Practice, Education, and Clinical Documentation Shared Governance Committee at our hospital. We are directly involved with educating our nursing staff in new competencies, just-in-time competencies, and annual competencies. … I love sharing knowledge and watching my fellow nurses grow. However, I still have a strong desire to be connected directly to our patients. This desire nudged me to begin a family nurse practitioner program. I will complete the program in July of 2016. My goal

is to then move on to get my DNP. I will still have the best of both worlds as clinician and educator.

Sabrina worked full time as a coordinator for hospice after attending the Clinical Nurse Educator Academy, but always wanted to return to academia:

> I have recently returned to the world of academia and am really pleased to be back! I recently returned to [community college] as a full-time assistant professor so I really am back to novice status ... learning a lot and loving it! ... I always knew I wanted to get back to teaching so lo and behold, I did it!
>
> You asked about a moment. For me it was the first time someone e-mailed me and referred to me as "Professor Sabrina." That was a thrill ... kind of silly I guess, but not to me. ... The work is hard and kind of never ending but I'm learning a lot and [this college] has defined itself as a "learning-centered" school so what's encouraged is consistent with many of the lessons you [the authors of this book] both taught and with my views and values related to education.

In Chapter 2, Donna tells of how it was joyful to watch smiles appear on her patients' faces when she made a difference for them. Eight years later, Donna is now an experienced clinical nurse educator at a community college and is making a difference for students. Their assessment of her skills as an excellent nurse educator reflect some of the concepts in this book: the importance of clinical expertise for teaching, excellent communication, helping the students to feel comfortable in their clinical learning environment, and celebrating their successes. Students wrote the following:

- Ms. Donna was a great clinical instructor! She made sure that all students feel comfort in actual clinical situations. If you take especially [an] OB class then you'd better have her as a clinical instructor! I really miss her a lot!
- She is a very inspiring professor. I learned a lot from my clinical with her and it was fun at the same time.
- She improved my assessment skills, showed me how to think and act like a nurse, and encouraged me when I was on the

correct course. She is very skilled as an OB nurse and I highly recommend her to anyone who wants to be a caring and skilled nurse.

- She gave to us the opportunity to learn. She motivated us to become a good nurse and to continue our education.

- Hands down the best professor in [this college]. She is very funny and she wants you to learn as much as you can. You must be receptive to learning because you will benefit from her mini lectures. You will hear her voice while taking your lecture exams because she tells you what you need to know. She must teach in lecture. We need a professor like her in OB!

- Ms. Donna is the best. She teaches you in a way that everything seems doable. She will prepare you to be a competent nurse and make it fun.

- I keep saying this again and again, this professor NEEDS TO TEACH in lecture! I learned A LOT from her, [more] than any OB lecture professor. If you're trying to sign up for her, GET HER NOW. QUICK! She's in demand! Also, she is so nice and helpful! I wish I could have her for med–surg too!!!

- Ms. Donna is an amazing instructor. I had her for med–surg clinical but her specialty is actually OB. I highly recommend her as a clinical instructor, especially if you are lucky enough to get her for maternal/fetal medicine. She will make you a great nurse, you will have fantastic assessment skills, and you will love learning. Two thumbs up!

Closing Thoughts

Stories present a unique way of describing, formulating, and reflecting upon experiences. They provide a range of perspectives that offer different and complementary insights to expand the theoretical information found in traditional textbooks (Baker, 2015). Evidence from stories is not generalizable, replicable, or subject to the stringent requirements of positivist research methodologies. Stories can, however, help us understand individualized perspectives that may not be accessed through traditional research and evidence bases. They help us come to understand aspects of persons' experiences that *they* feel are most relevant (Baker, 2015).

In addressing the problem of decontextualized knowledge, stories provide a context for learning through highlighting nuances of experience and drawing out elements of care that are important in nursing practice (Baker, 2015). As stated in the preface, "If stories come to you, care for them. And learn to give them away where they are needed" (Lopez, 1990, p. 48). Nurse clinicians who have shared their first-hand narratives here have provided a valuable context for helping us understand the fears and joys of transitioning from expert clinician to novice nurse educator. We hope future clinical nurse educators will continue to share their stories of making a difference for patients, colleagues, and students.

REFERENCES

Baker, C. (2015). Narrative in nursing practice, education and research. *Journal of Psychiatric and Mental Health Nursing*, 22, 1–2.

Benner, P., Sutphen, M., Leonard, V., & and Day, L. (2010). *Educating nurses: A call for radical transformation.* San Francisco, CA: Jossey-Bass.

Diekelmann, N. (2001). Narrative pedagogy: Heideggerian hermeneutical analysis of lived experiences of students, teachers and clinicians. *Advances in Nursing Science*, 23(3), 53–71.

Garlikov, R. (n.d.). The Socratic method. Teaching by asking instead of by telling. Retrieved from www.garlikov.com/Soc_Meth.html

Lopez, B. (1990). *Crow and Weasel.* San Francisco, CA: North Point Press.

Index

CPSIA information can be obtained
at www.ICGtesting.com
Printed in the USA
LVHW042042030320
648869LV00018B/585

9 780826 125989